Praise for Nancy Lynne Harris, M.A.

"I have worked with Nancy for many years. She is a great spiritual healer. She knows what it takes to heal permanently from a chronic problem as well as provide a short-term relief to the client. I would recommend her to anyone seeking to address a chronic or so-called incurable issue. She can help you diagnose the root cause of the problem. She helps heal from within unlike the modern day treatment which suppresses the symptoms."

Hemal Mehta, Computer Systems Expert,
U.S. Defense, Texas USA

"I'm writing to thank you so much. Working with you, for my daughter and myself, after years of counseling therapy, has been the most effective thing I have ever done to help my daughter. Life is much more pleasant at home. The energy is lighter for both of us. She is ready to face challenges in her life and resolve problems rather than running away, and her father and I are calmer and more at peace in our relationship with her. The work you do is simply amazing."

Margaret, Caring Mother, California USA

"Nancy is incredibly insightful and skillful at discovering and resolving those deep and often long-standing issues and blocks within us. Her treatments allowed me to move forward and start fully living again after I was stuck for 8 years of grieving after the devastating loss of a loved one. I trust her totally and recommend her highly. My quality of life was completely transformed, and I'm now a happy optimistic person embracing the life I was meant to live!"

Pam McLellan, www.WorkWithPam.com, Oregon USA

"The advancements you are making in your work are very exciting and inspirational! I want you to know how much I value you and your work and have enjoyed your workshops. I have received so many blessings from your healing work during my time of intense grief, and our musical adventures together."

Kalia Bethany, Musician and Life Coach,
www.KaliaBethany.com, Oregon USA

"I will never stop thanking you for everything you have done for my family, especially my children. For the moment, I can only ask God to watch over you and bless you much while I wait and find the opportunity to meet you personally and when that happens I do not want to leave you. Really! I love you very much. May God continue to bless you forever!"

Lupe, Caring Mother, California USA

"Best Christmas in my 66 years on this earth!! I carry the affirmation – I AM GODSPIRIT around with me. It is so unusual to not feel the pressure in my mind space. I woke up singing in my mind a little song, I LOVE ME, I LOVE ME, over and over. Thanks to you, I can use my God power and not believe I have to depend on something or someone outside of me to do it for me. Thank you so much for the exact WORDS to use!!! I am looking forward to the arrival of your next book in the mail. Thank you so much for being the caring and loving, powerful person YOU are!"

Love, light and blessings, Anna, Australia

MIRACLES
MASTER THE ART

Healing Medically Incurable Illness

NANCY LYNNE HARRIS, M.A.

GodSpirits United, LLC
Eugene, Oregon

Information on the Virtues adapted from the writings of William W. Walter, b. 1869 – d. 1941.

To protect the privacy of others, certain names and details have been changed.

Published and distributed by: GodSpirits United, LLC
www.GodSpiritsUnited.com

Publisher's Cataloging-in-Publication Data
provided by Five Rainbows Cataloging Services

Names: Harris, Nancy Lynne.
Title: Miracles master the art : healing medically incurable illness / Nancy Lynne Harris.
Description: Eugene, OR : GodSpirits United, 2016.
Identifiers: ISBN 978-0-9815-0464-3 (pbk.) | ISBN 978-0-9815-0463-6 (ebook)
Subjects: LCSH: Mind and body therapies. | Alternative medicine. | Mental healing. | Energy psychology. | Behavior modification. | Attitude (Psychology) | BISAC: BODY, MIND & SPIRIT / Healing / Prayer & Spiritual. | HEALTH & FITNESS / Healing.
Classification: LCC RC489.M53 H37 2016 (print) | LCC RC489.M53 (ebook) | DDC: 615.852/8—dc23.

ISBN: 978-0-9815-0463-6 (e-book) CreateSpace, Kindle, Kobo, Nook, iTunes, BookBaby
ISBN: 978-0-9815-0464-3 (tradepaper)
www.GodSpiritsUnited.com or www.Amazon.com
Cover and text design by: Mayapriya Long, www.Bookwrights.com
1st edition, April 2016
Manufactured in the United States of America

TO ALL THE PRECIOUS CHILDREN
OF THE WORLD WITH LOVE

ALSO BY NANCY LYNNE HARRIS, M.A.

Heal Yourself of Anything Example Glaucoma

ISBN: 978-0-9636-7812-6 (tradepaper)
ISBN: 978-0-9636-7815-7 (CD)

Consciously Overcome Mental Illness

ISBN: 978-0-9636-7816-4 (tradepaper)
ISBN: 978-0-9636-7817-1 (2-CD set)

How to Heal Your Hang-Ups – alcohol, depression, drug addiction

ISBN: 978-0-9815-0460-5 (CD)

Healing Alcoholism Invasion Revealed

ISBN: 978-0-9815-0461-2 (Kindle, Kobo, iTunes, Nook, BookBaby)
ISBN: 978-0-9815-0462-9 (tradepaper)

Available from www.GodSpiritsUnited.com or www.Amazon.com

CONTENTS

IMAGES AND CHARTS

ACKNOWLEDGMENT

It is with deep gratitude that I acknowledge Wonetta Abbeg from Springfield, Oregon, for her fine assistance in helping me set up this book on the computer in preparation for sending it to the book designer. Without her help, this achievement might not have been accomplished.

IN THE LIGHT

A radiant light is shining from me.
I fly with the eagles soaring above the earth.
I lie in the clouds
And harvest the dewdrops of heaven.
I dine with the Gods
and feast with the angels.
I am heaven bound in
Light energy and transformation,
a new creature at last.
I am Spirit.

~Nancy Lynne Harris

CHAPTER ONE

12 STEPS TO HEAL YOURSELF WITHOUT MEDICINE

It was 1980. When the call came in, I was presenting a jazz workshop for piano teachers in the farmlands of central Washington. My husband, Ray, was called to the phone. I continued presenting the workshop, wondering what was so important that someone was calling him while we were miles away from our home in Auburn, Washington.

When the workshop ended, we said our goodbyes and got into our car for the long drive home. Ray started the car, backed out a few feet, stopped, and looked at me with tears in his eyes. He said, "Oh, honey! That was Jeff on the phone." Jeff was our oldest son, just twenty years old.

Ray continued, "He said a policeman came to our home early this morning to say that Mike was killed in a car accident." Mike, our second child, had turned eighteen just eight days earlier. As we drove through the Washington countryside, now eager to get home, I tuned in to the news on the car radio, and we heard them announce the death of our son, Michael Alan Jones.

Michael was born in Frankfurt, Germany, while Ray was serving in the U.S. Army. It was an easy birth for me, mainly because I was in my mid-twenties. While I was still in the hospital, an Army doctor who specialized in ophthalmology came by to say he believed our baby might have something wrong with his eyes, and he wanted to see us in his office the following week. We complied, and the doctor confirmed that Michael was born with congenital glaucoma. The doctor explained that fluid was flowing into his eyes faster than it could flow out, which could cause excessive pressure on his optic nerve and lead to blindness. He also said that when the baby was old enough he would need to have surgery to save his sight.

When Michael reached the appointed age of eighteen months, we were living in military quarters at the Presidio of San Francisco, where another highly skilled ophthalmologist performed surgery twice on his eyes over a period of months. For the next eight years Michael was given daily eye drops and was taken to the doctor at regular intervals to have his eye pressure checked and prescriptions written for medicated eye drops.

Being the open-minded person that I am, I always felt there was a way for Michael to be healed, if only I could find it, in spite of the doctors who said he would always have glaucoma because they did not know how to heal it. When Ray's military service ended, we moved from the Bay Area to Santa Barbara, California, and "just happened" to move right across the street from a lady named Evelyn. I saw her out on her lawn one day, so I went over to meet my new neighbor. As we talked, I told her about Michael's glaucoma, and she told me she taught a class in healing, and that it was possible that Michael could be healed if we studied the course. I was ready to study anything if there was even a remote chance of healing, so we agreed.

The course she taught was written by a man named William Walter, who, through intensive reading and study, had healed himself of tuberculosis, and then developed this course to train other people in how to heal themselves of medically incurable illnesses. The course taught us that:

OUR THINKING CAUSES EVERYTHING THAT WE EXPERIENCE.

As time went on, using this approach, we began to have success in healing many things, like the common cold and the annual flu. After we had studied this course for two years, Ray and I went to Los Angeles to take the teachers' training. We both became certified teachers of Eschatology, the Science of Last Things. Then Ray accepted a position as a purchasing agent in San Jose, California, so once again we moved.

When Michael was nine years old, he still had glaucoma, was still being given daily prescription eye drops, and was still seeing an accredited ophthalmologist, now in the Bay Area, but I felt the time had come for us to take our stand for healing. I had just taken him in for his three-month pressure check, and with medication his eye pressure was under control. The next day I consciously chose to stop putting the medicated prescription drops in his eyes because I felt I had my thoughts in the right place to accomplish his healing.

Three months later I took Michael to the ophthalmologist for his checkup. The nurse took us into an examination room and asked me what time he had been given his drops that morning. I said, "I have not given him any drops for three months." She gave me a look of disbelief and noted that on his chart. When the doctor came into the room, he was angry. He said, "Why have you stopped the drops?" I simply said, "We did not do it ignorantly." The doctor was obviously shaken. He tried to calm down and proceeded to check Michael's eye pressure. Then he became quiet, and after a pause he said, "His pressure checks normal." I was elated, but I said nothing.

The doctor left the room briefly. When he returned, he said his colleague, also an ophthalmologist, was asking my permission to follow Michael's progress along with him from now on. I simply said "No." I knew that looking for glaucoma in my child's eyes could reproduce it. That was the last time Michael went to the ophthalmologist. His glaucoma had vanished.

What we learned in Eschatology is that our son's glaucoma was caused by *my feeling* of being pressured (controlled, domineered) by my mother-in-law, Coleen. She could not let go of her son Ray, my husband, even though we had been married for many years and had three children of our own. She wanted her own way and expected our obedience. I disliked her very much because of her constant intrusion and demands. Once I learned in Eschatology that she was the source of the pressure I was feeling that was causing Michael's glaucoma, I knew I had to stand against this woman and learn how to say NO to her, rather than allowing her to push me around any longer. I had to change the way I dealt with her. Always before it had been impossible for me to do this, because she was

"Mother" after all, and I was trying to be respectful, but it was way out of control. If we did not do what she wanted, she would remind us that we were supposed to honor our parents.

Soon my opportunity came to stand up to her. She called one afternoon and asked us to come for dinner that evening. I said, "No, thank you. We will not be able to come." That was a first for me, and it felt so good! She continued to ask and argue, and I continued to say "NO." So she hung up. About five minutes later she called back and asked me again the same question: "Will you come for dinner?" Again I said, "No, thank you." She continued to urge me, and said Father (her husband) might die soon, and this would be the last time we could be together. (She had used that excuse before.) I stuck to my guns and did not budge. She hung up. Five minutes later she called back for the third time in fifteen minutes. It was as if she had totally forgotten that I had said no already, so we went through it all over again. When we hung up from that third call, I felt triumphant and no longer felt pushed around. I had pushed back, and by changing my attitude in how I handled her demands, I had changed my on-going *feelings* of being pushed around by her. *My feelings* had reflected on my child's eyes as glaucoma, even while he was in my womb. I healed him of glaucoma by taking an action that changed the way *I felt*. I had allowed that woman to push me around for years, and now it was over. I had *reversed my feelings of being pressured. Now I felt in control.*

YOUR NEGATIVE FEELINGS CREATE YOUR ILLNESS. REVERSE YOUR FEELING TO GET YOUR HEALING.

My husband Ray and I enjoyed thirty-six years of marriage and raised a family of four children before we divorced in 1995.

Many years later it was the week before Christmas in 2007 when my phone rang one morning. My daughter Elizabeth was calling with some terrible news. She said, "Mother, are you sitting down?" I said "Yes." She said, "Jeff hanged himself." She was telling me that my oldest son, now forty-eight years old, was gone. Jeff had been an Eagle Scout as a teenager and exemplary in many other ways. At this point he was married with two teenaged daughters. No explanation was offered by my daughter as to why he had taken this action. I loved Jeff with all my heart, so I went into an intense state of grief and disbelief, and found it hard to think of anything else.

In March 2008, three months after Jeff's death, I had an appointment to have my hair cut that day, so I parked my car at the beauty shop, opened the car door and put my leg out to step down, only to find that my left hipbone had separated from my spine. I managed to get out of the car, but without the hipbone connected to the spine, my left leg bones turned sideways in my body with nothing to hold them in place. I could hardly walk at all, and the pain was intense. I chose not to go to a doctor because I had no interest in surgery, and I knew there was a way to heal myself spiritually if I could just figure it out.

From March to September, sometimes my bones seemed to be more in alignment, but at other times I could find no comfort in standing, sitting, or lying down, and walking was difficult. I talked to my body, my bones, and my hip. I told them I accepted no change in the perfect order of my body, and I expected complete healing. Even as a single person at this point in my life, I managed to drive my car, shop for groceries, teach piano, and take care of my daily needs. However, by September six months had gone by, and I was still in pain and had not made much progress toward healing at all.

In September 2008 I finally began to look at my feelings. I said to myself, "HOW DO I FEEL ABOUT LOSING ANOTHER SON?" (My son Michael had died in a car accident in 1980, eight days after his eighteenth birthday.) I said to myself, "I FEEL DISCONNECTED FROM MY SON." By consciously recognizing how I felt about this new tragedy, it told me the mistake in thought that I was making. Before that moment I had been lost in grief over losing Jeff. So at that point I began to think the opposite thought:

"NOTHING CAN SEPARATE ME FROM THE LOVE OF GOD."

I consciously *added* these words to my thinking and said them out loud over and over. Within three days of adding this new positive thought, I knew that my hip and leg bones were re-connecting. By April 2009 I was feeling very well, so I decided to go to Sacred Heart Medical Center in Eugene, Oregon for an x-ray. Later that same afternoon the technician's nurse called to say the doctor could find no evidence of any new or previous hip fracture of any kind. I had manifested a perfect painless healing. Some people would call that a miracle, but I knew I had consciously caused it to happen by intentionally reversing my feelings.

IF YOU THINK THE "RIGHT" COMBINATION OF POSITIVE WORDS, YOU CAN HEAL ALMOST ANYTHING.

Because of the tragic experiences I have had in my life and the profound ways I have found to overcome them, at one point I asked the Powers-That-Be (which I call Spirit) to let me serve. I was then spiritually guided into training with The Four Winds Society that offers the world's most extensive professional training in energy healing, founded by Dr. Alberto Villoldo. Now, as a graduate of that program, I am trained as a Shaman in the tradition of the Inca of the Americas, and I love to do this work. As an energy healer and spiritual teacher, I founded my own company, GodSpirits United, LLC, to teach people how to heal themselves of medically incurable illnesses.

As children, most of us are trained to believe that when we are sick, someone else is supposed to fix us. We go to the doctor; we fill the prescription; we take the pills; we might have surgery; and then maybe we will get well and maybe we won't. But that is our mindset, whether or not it works. We are so brainwashed with medical remedies and the constant bombardment of our thinking from watching television commercials that sell medicines that we sometimes forget there are better ways to heal ourselves.

The doctor hopes to heal you by adding drugs to your blood chemistry. An energy healer heals you by removing the negative energy that causes your illness and tells you that finding a positive way to think about your problem will automatically improve your blood chemistry. A surgeon operates to remove a tumor, but leaves the negative energy that caused the tumor inside your body because he cannot see it (energy is invisible). An energy healer removes the negative energy that causes the tumor without surgery. In energy healing, there is never any cutting on your body. Even in addictions, things that are invasive (like demons or other entities) are painlessly removed using crystals. A doctor uses machines like CAT scanners and x-rays to see inside your physical body. An energy healer communicates with spirit guides and reads your energy using his or her chakras to see what your problem is. Your chakras are a natural part of your energy body.

It is a proven scientific fact that everything is energy. You are made of Creative Light Energy that is temporarily housed in and around your current physical body. The energy you are made of is controlled by your feelings and attitudes. Positive thoughts and feelings about yourself move your energy toward positive experiences, and negative thoughts and feelings about yourself move your energy toward negative experiences. The way you think and the choices you make control the organs in your body and regulate your blood chemistry. Your blood, cells, bodily tissues, and skin are all controlled by the way you think and feel, especially about yourself. If you do not like what you are experiencing, you have the option to change the way you think to something more positive.

Thinking is an exact science, and we are given no training in it at all as we grow up. Specific illnesses are caused by thinking specific words. The words you think are caused by the feelings you feel and the attitudes you choose to entertain. When your feelings are very strong in a negative way, to protect your health you have to choose which attitudes you're going to support–the feelings that will eventually make you sick or the opposite positive feelings that will keep you well. No one thinks in your mind but you, so your health is always your own choice.

The first and foremost thought that needs to be corrected for healing is your attitude about yourself. If you are hating yourself, even subconsciously, and using your negative words and feelings to berate yourself for any reason, you will have a hard time being successful in life or in healing your illness. If you find fault with yourself and with other people and blame them for your problems, you need to realize that finding fault is an extremely negative way to think and will create faults in your own body if continued. You have to begin to monitor your thinking moment by moment and be willing to think something positive and wholesome, if you want to experience a positive and wholesome life.

SELF-CORRECTION IS THE KEY TO HEALING MEDICALLY INCURABLE ILLNESS.

12 STEPS TO HEAL YOURSELF WITHOUT MEDICINE

The following twelve questions were designed to help you identify your own negative feelings that have caused the illness you want to overcome and to help you identify the opposite positive feeling words you need to think to reverse your illness for healing. Be sure you write down your answers in a special notebook for easy reference and deep contemplation and improvement at any time.

1. Write down the date when your illness began. What disturbing thing occurred in your life shortly before your illness appeared? You may not have linked whatever it was to your illness, but illnesses do not just pop out of thin air. To cause an illness, this occurrence was something you FELT deeply about, and your feeling was negative. What happened? What was this disturbance?
2. Exactly how did you FEEL about what happened? Why did you not like it? What word(s) would best describe your negative FEELINGS? Sum up your feelings in one or two precise words.
3. Use a dictionary or thesaurus to find the EXACT OPPOSITE POSITIVE WORD (the antonym) to the way this upsetting event or troublesome person made you FEEL. Be scientific in selecting this word.
4. How did you physically react to this situation? How did you cope? What did you do?
5. How long after the event did your illness appear? What were your symptoms?

6. What organ or organs in your body does this illness affect?
7. What is the medical name for your illness?
8. What negative things (beliefs) did the doctor tell you about the illness that you need to stop believing to make your healing possible? You cannot believe that you HAVE an illness and NOT HAVE IT at the same time.
9. How does this illness make your body feel? How would you describe your pain or discomfort?
10. Begin to reprogram your thinking by canceling the negative FEELING word(s) you identified in number two above. Say to yourself (your Creative Light Energy) repeatedly, "NO MORE (your negative feelings words)." Say "I DISPEL (your negative words)." *Dispel* means "to scatter or clear away." Imagine a mental trap shoot to see yourself blowing up these negative words in your mind.
11. Begin to claim and support the opposite positive word(s) as true. Think more about the positive way you DO want your health to be rather than continuing to think that you HAVE a health problem. If you want the problem to change, you have to change the way you think about it. You are made of Creative Light Energy that will give you exactly what you believe to be true. HOLD the positive word from number three above in your mind all day every day until you get what you want. Be relentless in thinking these positive words if you want your blood chemistry to change. When you are thinking the new positive word(s) 51 percent of the time, your health will automatically shift and your illness will vanish. Say, "NOW I FEEL (exact opposite positive FEELING word)."

12. Reversing an illness is much like covering an overdraft at the bank. When you are on the negative side of zero, you have to deposit a little more to cover the overdraft charge to get your bank balance back on the positive side. To get well, you must break your habit of allowing your negative feelings to control you or take you down. No matter what negative event has happened, to protect your health you must choose to think high-quality positive words like GRATITUDE, INSPIRATION, HARMONY, STRENGTH, ENDURANCE, JOY, COURAGE, PATIENCE, PERFECT, PURITY, and most important of all, SELF-LOVE. Add these good words to your thinking intentionally and daily. Your health will exactly reflect your degree of success in improving the way you think, especially about yourself, and your willingness to stop supporting any of your old negative feelings. Say repeatedly,

EVERY DAY IN EVERY WAY MY LIFE GETS BETTER.

Illness of all kinds is caused by the accumulation of negative energy in your mind and body. This negative energy can be cleaned out with energy treatments, but you need to become a positive thinker to keep from reloading yourself with more negative energy. Throw out your old negative attitudes. Once you begin to work on analyzing and reversing your negative feelings and monitoring and correcting your current feelings, your health will begin to improve automatically.

As long as you believe that you HAVE an illness, you will continue to have it. You are programming the energy you are made of every moment, so you have to learn to change your program if you want your health to change. You are not trained to think of yourself as energy that is programmable, but that is exactly what you are. Every thought you think is creating your current program, so keep your thinking all positive from now on, and you will have no illness. Your energy is yours to control.

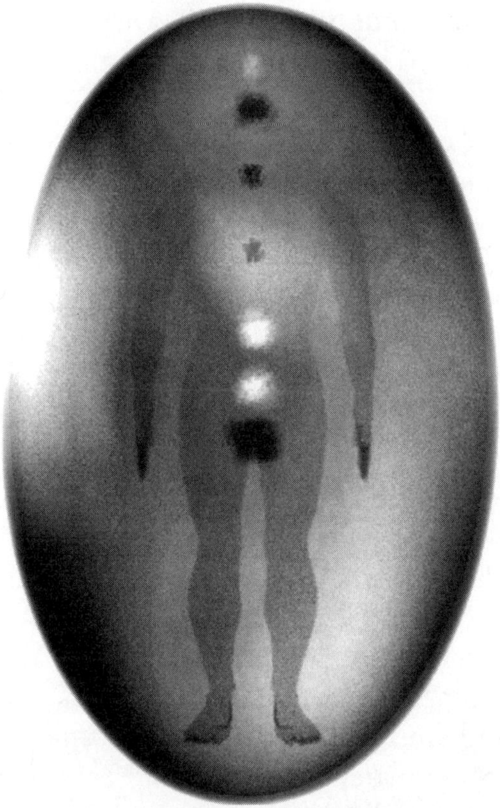

GODSPIRIT–MY AURA

CHAPTER TWO

THE POWER OF WORDS – USING WORDS AS MEDICINE

Have you ever had an illness that medicine could not heal? You know there are many illnesses that are not medically healable, even if you take the medicine for the rest of your life. Dr. James Marcum, a practicing cardiologist, says he is the first medical doctor to prove that the number one cause of death in America is *medications*. He believes in giving non-pharmacological methods to improve the body's blood chemistry. His book is called *Medicines That Kill*.

In spiritual healing we study techniques that work perfectly when they are used correctly, but these techniques are not commonly known. Even after you study spiritual healing, you stand in the way of your own success because your old thought habits and beliefs die hard in your mind. Your old ways will fight with the new techniques you're trying to use.

To study parts of your mind that you use all the time, without consciously thinking about it, we're going to take a journey. You may want to turn out the lights, or put on a blindfold, or just close your eyes. When you are ready, begin to imagine that you are on the beach on Maui, Hawaii. There you are, sitting in a comfortable lawn chair, relaxing and watching the breakers roll in. You feel the warm sun shining down on you, and it feels so good. You don't have a care in the world. The sky is like the most beautiful painting you ever saw, and the ocean is green and blue, turquoise and purple, tranquil and gorgeous. It looks almost unreal.

Now, with your eyes still closed, let's rise a little higher and think about what you just did. To observe yourself on Maui, you projected a vision on the *mental screen* of your mind. This mental screen is the *face* or *surface* of your deep mind. You can *project* visions, words, and feelings from **without-in** onto this screen, like we just did, or you can *observe* visions, words, and feelings that arise from the depth of your *deep* mind and come from **within-out**, like your dreams and inspirations, so this is a two-way screen, with your thoughts going in and out.

If you think about water, it always has a surface, whether it's in a fishbowl or an ocean, and it always has a deeper part. To imagine yourself on Maui, you were using the face or surface of your mind. We were not going into the deep mind. We have to learn to pay attention to our thinking and work consciously on the face or surface to change troublesome things in our deep mind that can cause us to be ill.

Now I want you to project a new vision onto your mental screen. This is an exercise that will open your mind to receive new information. Imagine a big circle that looks like the face of a clock. The little hand is pointing straight up toward high noon and cannot move. The big hand is pointing at the number 1, slightly to the right of high noon. The space between the two hands is bright green, indicating that your mind is open five degrees. The rest of the circle is black. I will ask you a question, and the big hand on your clock will begin to move around the clock to answer the question. Watch to see where the big hand stops. Then mentally take hold of it and move it clockwise, clear on around the clock, until both hands are pointing straight up at high noon, and the entire circle turns bright green. Are you ready? The question to ask yourself is: How open is my mind?

Where did the big hand stop before you moved it on around the clock? That is how open-minded you were a moment ago. Your mind is now completely open to receive new information. In this exercise, you have been working on the face or surface of your mind. This is where you work to shift or reverse energy to heal an illness. Now you can open your eyes.

In my training as an energy healer with The Four Winds Society, I learned that the Inca in Peru could shapeshift their bodies at will into jaguars or falcons and back again. Jesus and the Inca were both masters at controlling the same substance–Spirit or Creative Light Energy. Jesus would mentally *send His word* to heal people long distance. Why did Jesus *send His word* rather than a medical prescription or a diet or exercise plan? He "sent" what he understood controls and shifts Spirit or Creative Light Energy, which is:

WORDS–
THE MOST POWERFUL HEALER OF ALL.

In the beginning was the Word,
and the Word was with God,
and ***the Word WAS God.***

John 1:1

This means,

AS GOD, *WORDS* HAVE THE POWER TO SHIFT THE CREATIVE ENERGY!

Words ARE God! Why have we missed this for so long? You know the expression "I just did it without thinking." Well, it's time for us to stop thinking without thinking.

Jesus could read energy at any distance, so He instantly knew which negative word (or words) the sick person was thinking to create the illness. By sending positive words into their mental space to reverse the negative words they were thinking, Jesus shifted the energy in their bloodstream to positive and healed the person instantly. What does this mean?

THE WORDS YOU THINK CONTROL YOUR BLOOD CHEMISTRY.

So what healing requires is changing a negative word to a positive word in your mind. You have the ability to do this. If, at that point, all your negative beliefs about the illness come in to fight with your positive words and you buy into it, then you will prevent yourself from getting well. Healing yourself requires being willing to change negatives to positives on your mental screen and letting go of your negative beliefs. Once you focus a new positive word onto your mental screen, you have to know how to *send it into your bloodstream*. This is easy. Let's practice that right now.

Close your eyes. Project the word LOVE onto your mental screen so you can see the letters clearly. Now *send* that word LOVE into your own bloodstream with your intention. Energy healing is very intentional. Feel the word LOVE flowing all around in your body. Now let's send another word. Project and visualize the word STRONG onto your mental screen. Now *send* the word STRONG into your heart with your intention. Notice how that feels. Next, visualize the word JOY on your mental screen. *Send* the word JOY into your lungs. Keep these good words going in your mind every day to keep yourself well. Now open your eyes.

The indigenous people of Peru known as the Q'ero are the bloodline descendants of the high priests of the Inca. They say, **"WORDS ARE LIVING BEINGS."**

My logo for GodSpirits United, LLC, is a picture of my aura, my luminous energy field, photographed several years ago with a special software program. Everyone has an aura. It is a permanent part of your energy body that stores what you think and believe to be true like a filing cabinet. If you could see a picture of your aura, you would notice that the Light you see is *not shining on you*. Your auric light is *your God Light shining from you*. YOU are made of Conscious Living Light Energy that breathes the body temple that you currently indwell. You are a GodSpirit, if you will. You are MUCH GREATER than you think you are, and much more powerful than you can even imagine.

Know ye not that ye are the temple of God,
And that the Spirit of God dwells in you?

I Cor. 3:16

Quantum physics has proved that everything is energy. You live and move and have your being because you are made of Living Light Energy. Everything is vibrating Light. The problem is that you do not think of yourself as Light Energy. You think you are the butcher, the baker, the candlestick maker, the mother, the father, the daughter, the son. We play many roles. We even think we are human, but we are NOT human. Webster defines *human* as "higher than the animals but lower than God." We need to throw that definition away. You, as Creative Light Energy, are the highest substance in existence, descended from the family of Spirit. If Eve was made from Adam's rib, Adam was made from God's rib, and so were you, because we beget each other. Your origin was Spirit, the only substance there ever was or ever will be. It's time to re-evaluate and greatly elevate the way you think about your "Self."

You, as an individual portion of Living Light Energy called Spirit, need to learn how to control your individual portion of the elemental substance you are made of. Your own Living Energy is programmed and controlled by your feelings, your words, and your actions.

While I lived in Santa Barbara, California, I had a friend and client named Esther, who was in her mid-seventies. She would hire me to give her energy treatments to clean the negative energy out of her auric field, because she believed she was going blind. Once this old negative energy is cleaned out, you need to stay positive and not reload yourself with the negative feelings and beliefs that were just cleaned out. But Esther would always finish her treatments by saying out loud, "I'm going blind," so she would instantly reload her auric field with her negative belief, and that is exactly what happened to her. By the time she passed away, she was completely blind. You have to think in the positive way you want your energy to flow, rather than the negative way things seem to be going, because your energy is always listening to the programs you are creating and will always comply with your heart feelings and beliefs.

If you concentrate on a negative word 51 percent or more of the time, you will create and experience a negative outcome. If you concentrate on a positive word 51 percent or more of the time, you will create and experience a positive outcome. You can always change your mind, so nothing hinders you from creating what you want. You must keep your negative feelings under control if you want to experience a positive outcome.

ENERGY SHIFTS IN PROPORTION TO THE WEIGHT OF YOUR POSITIVE OR NEGATIVE BELIEFS.

Earlier I told the story of how my left hipbone disconnected from my spine in March 2008, three months after the suicide of my son Jeff. I want to explain more clearly how I healed myself. I chose not to go to a doctor in spite of the pain I was in, because I knew there was a spiritual way to heal myself, and I was determined to find it. At the time this happened, I was divorced after thirty-six years of marriage and lived alone, so walking was a vital necessity for me. I was not interested in surgery to reconnect my bones, because I knew there was a better way, and I knew I could heal myself if I could find the right words to think. I also knew from past experience that praying for healing in the religious sense and leaving it up to God was too risky and uncertain. You never know how that will turn out. I knew I could use positive words to heal myself, but I had not yet understood what the positive word was that I needed to think to cause my bones to reconnect so I could walk normally without pain once again.

In September 2008 I had finally waded through my grief enough to ask myself the question "HOW DO I *FEEL* ABOUT LOSING *ANOTHER* SON?" (I had already lost my son Michael in a car accident in 1980.) The answer came to me instantly. "*DISCONNECTED* from my son! That's how I feel." *Disconnected* was the word I needed to reverse to accomplish my healing. By consciously recognizing my negative feelings about this tragedy, I understood the mistake in thought that I was making. So at that point I began to think the opposite thought:

"NOTHING CAN SEPARATE ME FROM THE LOVE OF GOD."

By consciously *adding* these positive words to my thinking and saying them out loud over and over, my hip and leg bones began to reconnect and heal. Within three days of adding this new positive thought, I knew I was getting better. By the time I went in for an x-ray in April 2009, I had manifested a perfect painless healing, and the x-ray technician said he could find no evidence of any new or previous hip fracture of any kind. So how can *you* learn to do this?

THREE STEPS TO HEAL YOURSELF

1. Identify your negative feeling as a *word*, and write it down. Ask yourself, "How do I *feel* about what happened?"

2. Reverse your feeling intentionally by *adding* the opposite positive word (the antonym) to your thinking. I said, "NOTHING CAN SEPARATE ME." I could also have said, "I AM CONNECTED," to reverse my feeling of being *disconnected*.
3. Your body will automatically begin to reflect the change once you begin to give the positive command to your energy, and you will know you are getting well. The trick is to correctly identify *the* negative feeling word so you can consciously reverse it in your thinking to get the positive result you want in your health, your bank account, or your life (whatever you are working on). Until you identify your negative feeling accurately and reverse it consciously in your thoughts, you will continue to manifest your illness or other problem. (There are some illnesses that may require special energy treatments to remove invisible negative elements that can prevent an illness from leaving if they are not dealt with first, *e.g.*, karma, curses.)

When you are treating yourself, you don't have to say "I AM" COURAGEOUS, because *"I AM" is what you are.* The positive word alone is enough to heal you. You are the Living Energy and the thinker giving instructions to your own portion of Living Spirit. Positive words, like *empowered, strong,* and *life*, heal your heart. Inspirational words, like *encouraged* and *joy,* heal your lungs, and we will talk more about specific words that govern your organs. Your body always follows your own programming.

One day while I was married, my husband, Ray, came home from work limping. I asked him what was wrong, and he said he had a bad pain in his knee. I told him to go into a dark closet when the pain was hurting and look inward to see what negative word was appearing on his mental screen. After a while he came out of the closet and said he saw the word "failure" on his screen. He then told me that when he was a child his dad told him his brother Dick would be a success and he, Ray, would be a failure in life. That negative mis-teaching from childhood was still haunting him. I told him to reverse the word "failure" in his mind by actively thinking that he was a great success, which he actually was. He did this, and in a short time the pain in his knee disappeared.

When you feel a pain in your body and you don't know what is causing it, you can discover the exact negative word you need to reverse by going into a closet or a dark place ***when your pain is hurting*** and by looking inward at your mental screen. The negative word that is causing your pain will have risen to the surface of your mind where you can see it. Once you see what that word is, reverse the word to get your healing.

Your mind is a container full of *WORDS*, so you have to pay attention to the quality of words you are filling it with. Your body is like a thermometer that reflects the majority of the positive or negative words you think, so the higher the quality, refinement, and purity in your thinking, the greater health, wealth, and happiness you will manifest in your body and in your life.

One of the worst things you can ever do is to swear at yourself or to swear at God. It fills the chambers of your soul with psychic manure. Then you wonder why your life is not going well. You don't want to attract people into your life who will swear at you and abuse you, so do not treat yourself that way. No one but you thinks in your mind, so pay attention to what you are creating with the words you are thinking and speaking. Never say things like "I could just kick myself," because even that is self-abuse.

The Creative Energy that breathes your body is like a loving parent who wants to give you whatever you want. It responds specifically to your self-talk, your inner visions, and your heart's motive. It hears every thought you think and every word you speak, because *IT IS YOU*. Your challenge is in learning to ***use*** your Creative Energy consciously, rather than believing it's something "out there somewhere" you worship or pray to.

The Q'ero of Peru say that praying to an unseen benevolent power to move the Creative Energy for you is *not* the correct way to move it. Saying "Please, God, hear my prayer" is not the way to get the results you want. Like Jesus, the Q'ero *command* the energy to move. They say "HAMPE RAIN" or "HAMPE PEACE," and I have seen and heard them do this. They are emphatic in the way they say it. *Hampe* means "ENERGY HEALING" or "COME" as a command in the Q'echuan language.

This is exactly the way Jesus healed. When His friend Lazarus died, Jesus cried with a loud voice, *Lazarus, come forth* (John 11:43), and Lazarus opened his eyes. To the man lame with palsy, Jesus said, *Arise, take up your bed, and go into your house.* (Luke 4:23). To us, he says, *Physician, heal thyself!* (Luke 4:23)

It's time that we learn to command the energy ourselves using positive words that our body responds to, and stop expecting someone else to heal us with pills, surgeries, and other artificial and harmful means. We can control the Creative Energy by commanding it with action words to *MOVE NOW*. If you doubt your ability to make the Creative

Energy move the way you want it to move, it's because you don't understand yourself as energy, and because you've never been trained to monitor your thinking. If you doubt that you have the ability to make the Creative Energy move with your thoughts, your self-doubt will prevent it from moving the way it would respond if you believed in yourself even a little. The Creative Energy always knows what you are thinking, because it is what you are, so it is vital for your own well-being that you learn how to control what you are made of. Your body will always register how well you are doing.

SIX STEPS TO GAIN CONTROL OF YOURSELF

1. **Monitor** your thinking all of the time.
2. **Reverse** your negative self-talk instantly the moment you notice it.
3. **Add** positive words to your thinking consciously.
4. **Believe** in yourself a lot more than you have in the past.
5. **Understand** that your positive or negative attitudes control your blood chemistry.
6. **Think** of yourself as Creative Light Energy capable of everything to the extent you believe in yourself.

Have you ever heard someone say, "I have cancer, and we're going to fight it"? Never fight with a disease. A disease is always a negative. The more attention you give to it, the more power you give it. Stop claiming that you have anything that you don't want. Remember, it's just a negative feeling word that you thought that caused the illness to manifest itself, (in the case of cancer, the feeling of resentment), and a feeling can always be reversed. What does your thesaurus say is the opposite of resentment? My thesaurus says: "affection, amity, concord, harmony, pleasure, endearment, patience, happiness, geniality, enthusiasm, compliance, good humor."

**ATTITUDES ARE EVERYTHING.
THEY CREATE YOUR LIFE.**

If you learn to reverse or shift the Creative Energy that you are made of, it gives you power over your body, your bloodstream, and your health. By being willing to change your negative feeling words to positive feeling words in your own mind, you'll be doing it right, and you'll move out of the role of victim into the role of *MASTER*.

Now stand up and close your eyes. Imagine that you are standing in the middle of your mental screen with your Creative Light Energy *shining from you–not on you–but from you*. Now say out loud,

**"I AM CREATIVE LIGHT ENERGY,
THE MOST POWERFUL SUBSTANCE
IN EXISTENCE."**

Then say it again even louder:

**"I AM CREATIVE LIGHT ENERGY,
THE MOST POWERFUL SUBSTANCE
IN EXISTENCE."**

Notice how good that makes your body feel.

LET YOURSELF BE GREAT, BECAUSE YOU ARE.

Now you can open your eyes.

THE WORD WAS GOD.

John 1:1

ADD high-level positive words to your thinking every day to help maintain the positive chemical balance in your bloodstream. Correlate words to the day of the month. For days 27–31, ADD your own positive words.

1.	A	Able	Abundance	Accepted
		Accomplished	Acquitted	Ageless
		Alive	Ample	Angels
		Appeased	Appreciated	Approving
		Ascension	Assured	Awesome
2.	B	Balanced	Beatitude	Beautifu
		Believe	Bending	Better
		Blessed	Bliss	Buoyant
3.	C	Calm	Capable	Caring
		Celebrating	Centered	Changing
		Cherished	Circulating	Clarity
		Clean	Comfortable	Compassionate
		Confident	Connected	Contented
4.	D	Dancing	Deep	Delighted
		Deserving	Desirable	Devoted
		Dignity	Divine	
5.	E	Ease	Ecstatic	Elated
		Empowered	Encouraged	Endowed

		Enduring	Enjoying	Enthusiastic
		Energetic	Enlightened	Enriched
		Essential	Eternal	Excelling
6.	F	Fabulous	Faithful	Fantastic
		Favorable	Fearless	Fine
		Flexible	Focused	Forgiving
		Fortunate	Free	Friendly
		Fulfilled	Fun	
7.	G	Gaining	Generous	Gentle
		Giving	Glad	Glorious
		Godly	Good	Graceful
		Gracious	Grand	Grateful
		Grounded	Growing	Guided
8.	H	Happy	Harmonious	Healing
		Healthy	Hearty	Heaven
		Helpful	Holy	Honest
9.	I	Ideal	Imagination	Immortal
		Impunity	Income	Ingenuity
		Innocent	Inspired	Integrity
		Intelligent	Intentional	Interesting
		Intuition	Investing	Invoke
10.	J	Jovial	Joyful	Just
11.	K	Kind	Knowledgeable	

12.	L	Laughing	Learning	Living
		Lifting	Light	Loving/Loved
		Loyal	Lucky	
13.	M	Magnificent	Majestic	Marvelous
		Meditative	Mental	Merciful
		Mindful	Miraculous	
14.	N	Natural	Needed	New
15.	O	Open-minded	Optimistic	Opulent
16.	P	Paradise	Patient	Peaceful
		Perfect	Persistent	Playful
		Pleasurable	Plenty	Praising
		Progressing	Prosperous	Positive
		Powerful	Precious	Protected
17.	Q	Quality	Quantity	Quiet
18.	R	Radiant	Reasonable	Recognized
		Refreshed	Regenerated	Rejoicing
		Relaxed	Relieved	Renewed
		Resting	Rich	Righteous
19.	S	Sacred	Safe	Sanctified
		Sane	Satisfied	Secure
		Self	Sensible	Serene
		Serving	Seeing	Sincere

		Singing	Smiling	Special
		Spiritual	Splendid	Soft
		Soulful	Stable	Stamina
		Strong	Sweet	Substance
		Successful	Sufficient	Supported
20.	T	Talented	Tender	Thankful
		Thinking	Thriving	Thoughtful
		Tranquil	Transcending	Transmuting
		Triumphant	Trusting	Truthful
21.	U	Unafraid	Understanding	Unlimited
22.	V	Valuable	Vibrant	Victorious
		Virtuous	Vision	Vital
23.	W	Wealthy	Well	Whole
		Wise	Wonderful	Worthy
24.	X	Excellent	Exceptional	Exuberant
25.	Y	Young	Youthful	
26.	Z	Zealous		

CHAPTER THREE

LOVING YOUR S. E. L. F. – SCIENTIFICALLY EVOLVING LIFE FORCE

There is an old wives' tale that says "Loving yourself is selfish and conceited." This fallacious belief has been passed down through the generations for centuries, and it is causing more dysfunction and poverty on earth than anyone can imagine. It's time for this to change.

We do not always understand that we are spiritually controlled, but we are, from the moment we are born until the moment we die, and beyond, through built-in controls. We may not be aware that the words we think and speak control the organs in our body, but they do every moment of the day. We also may not know that the positive and negative words that we think regulate and control our blood chemistry and our health, but they do. It's time to realize that the old wives' tale that says loving yourself is selfish and conceited does more damage and hurts more people than just about any other misconception on earth.

If you want to guarantee that your children will grow

up to be alcoholics, drug addicts, prostitutes, mentally ill, or die of Alzheimer's, just teach them while they are still young not to love themselves. The world is already full of people like this. We go on and on harming ourselves without meaning to with this pernicious teaching. And then we cry and grieve and wonder why we have no mental peace. We thought we were doing our best.

Years ago I had a friend named Joe who sold digital pianos out of his home. I used to play background jazz piano for parties, and I had a gig coming up, so I drove over to Joe's house to rent a keyboard. When I arrived, he said his wife, Kathy, was suffering from depression. They belonged to a church that taught their practitioners to give all their love to God, because their belief was that God is everything and we are nothing, and to love one's self is selfish and conceited.

Kathy had followed these instructions to the letter. She had given all her love to God literally, just draining herself, and, as a result, she was quite mentally ill. Her doctor had given her some pills, but Joe and Kathy never suspected that her depression was caused from her conscious intention to strip herself of love. Without love for herself, she was in spiritual darkness, in spite of her good intentions, through adherence to fallacious teachings by well-meaning people who grossly misunderstood what they were doing. The Old Testament tells us to love God, but the problem arises when we do not identify our Self with what God is.

I, too, was taught not to love myself as a child. When I was about eight years old, my mother, Grace, and I were dusting the dining room one day and having a conversation about whom we could love. I asked her directly if it was okay for me to love myself. Mother said, "Oh, no, you just love other people." She said that loving yourself is conceited. So I grew up trying hard to love other people while withholding love from myself. My mother's unintentional mis-teaching that day led to serious problems for me as a young married woman. Without love for myself, I found nothing at all to sustain me or help me withstand the shock when my eighteen-year-old son Michael was instantly killed in a car accident. My counselor at the time said my mother had set me up for depression by teaching me not to love myself.

Depression in its darkest form is a state of mind you never want to experience. The opposite of self-love is self-hatred, and self-hatred results in an atmosphere of mental hell. There are millions of people on earth who have not learned to love themselves, or were taught not to, so to get through the tough times in life they may feel their only options are alcohol, drugs, or suicide.

In a state of depression, you may or may not find the help that you need in the usual places you expect to find it, no matter how many medications you swallow or how well-meaning your doctor or counselor may be. Unfortunately, medically-trained people may think you're just imagining the nightmare you're going through, which will not be beneficial to you at all. Our medically-based mental health system does its best, but medications still fail to heal millions of dysfunctional people every year. Eventually, through my own reasoning and studies, I came to understand what was causing my depression, and I was able to heal myself.

THINKING SELF-LOVE CONSTANTLY IS THE ONLY WAY TO GET WELL.

Coming from a place of love for your SELF, you brighten your own auric light and thereby cause the disturbances in your mind to gradually diminish. The more you say positive loving things to yourself in your self-talk, the better your life will become in every way. When you have filled yourself with love first, you have a lot more love to give to other people. This old wives' tale, that loving yourself is conceited, needs to end forever, so we can improve our relationship with our Self and with one another, and watch dysfunction disappear from our world as a result.

After I recovered from depression, I did some research on the meaning of the word "conceit," since my mother had said loving yourself is conceited. According to *Webster's Dictionary*, *conceit* means, "Endowed with intelligence and imagination, favorably minded, thinking, mental activity, high estimation, ingenious, aptitude, discernment, originality, and resourcefulness." Synonyms are "clever, idea, concept, judgment, self-love, understand, self-esteem, and admiration." The opposite word, *conceitless,* means "lack of understanding." A synonym for *conceitless* is "ignorance." You can easily verify the positive meaning of the word "conceit" by looking it up in your own dictionary. It's time for us to learn what "conceit" really means, and be proud to love ourselves openly.

Many people go through their entire life without ever consciously recognizing their own being, their own conscious SELF. They just look out at other people, believing that "out there" in the world is reality. Actually, just the opposite is true. What is going on in your own mind is projecting what you are experiencing in your body and in the world, whether or not you are aware of it. If you don't pay attention to your SELF and learn to monitor what you're thinking, you're missing the main event.

My dear mother, Grace, lived only in perception. What she could see looking outward was all she knew, and her mother probably taught her not to love herself. In 2007, Mother died of Alzheimer's after a ten-year illness. In Alzheimer's you lose your SELF. You don't know who you are or who your children are. Your brain disintegrates, and you are unable to function normally. There are more than forty-five million people in the world today with Alzheimer's and one-in-nine Americans over age sixty-five, and that number is growing. I am convinced that a lack of *conceit*, which is a lack of Self-Love, causes Alzheimer's.

Not loving yourself breaks the great spiritual commandment:

Thou shalt love thy neighbor as thyself. Rom. 13:9

The Self part gets ignored in common practice.

Love your-Self as your neighbor.

Now we're going to do an exercise to learn more about the inner workings of your mind. You need to have a blindfold handy, but don't put it on yet. When we look outward, we need light to help us see, but when we look inward, we have to use our inner sense of vision to see in the dark. To begin this exercise, I want you to look at something far away, like a cloud or an airplane. If you're in a room, just look at something on the other side of the room. Now look at the palm of your hand. This is often where people stop looking, sometimes even during meditation, without realizing that we can reverse our vision and go right on seeing by looking inward. Now, either put on the blindfold or just close your eyes.

We're going to explore your inner mental space (the screen of your mind). Begin to look inward into the darkness until you can see what looks like the stars in the night sky. You don't have to imagine the stars or the sky; just let them appear. They're already naturally there. Sometimes it takes two or three minutes to see them clearly. When they come into focus, imagine that you're looking at a little spot of light that's down at the very bottom center of your mental space. This is a spot of bright light that you control. It's like it's down there on the floor of your mind.

Once you see the light shining there clearly in the darkness, begin to move it to the right as far as it will go, always staying within your own individual mental space. When you feel you have moved it as far as it will go to the right, begin to move the spot of light upward and just notice what you sense. How high can you go? Is there a ceiling in here? How far up can you move it before it begins to pull toward the left? Just keep moving it and see what happens. As you go across the top of your mental space, you'll come to a place where the light will begin to descend down the left side. Just keep moving it down, and when you reach the bottom again, slowly bring the light back to the place at the bottom center where you started. You've made a giant circle around the whole inner perimeter of your individual mental space. At this point, turn out the spot of light you've been moving around, so your inner space is completely dark except for the stars in the night sky.

Now we're going to use remote viewing to look at something far away. Imagine that you are in an airplane that's about to land in Paris. You disembark and get into a limousine that takes you directly to the Eiffel Tower. You get out of the limousine and look up at the elevator that's taking people up and down on the tower. Right now the elevator is coming down. Now look carefully. How many people do you see in the elevator right now? At the count of six, come back into this room, take off your blindfold, and open your eyes. 1-2-3-4-5-6. How many people did you see in the elevator?

The Kogi Indians of Guatemala raise their babies that are destined to be tribal leaders in near darkness for the first nine years of their lives, so they will have highly developed inner vision. These children grow up to be the medicine people, the wise ones, who communicate with Spirit and move energy at will because they can see what's going on in the Spirit world. For those of us who were not raised in the dark, we can still learn to look into our mind, monitor our thinking, and exercise control over our life.

George Lamsa, who was of Assyrian descent, has translated the Holy Bible from the original Aramaic text into English. Aramaic was the language Jesus spoke. As a native of ancient biblical lands, where he lived until World War I, Mr. Lamsa was uniquely fitted for this task, because his people retained biblical customs and Semitic culture which had perished virtually everywhere else. His background enabled him to recover much of the meaning lost in other translations of the Scriptures.

Interpreting the use of the word "me" in the Bible can be thought-provoking. For instance, Mr. Lamsa's translation of Exodus 20:3 is:

You shall have no other Gods except me.

The King James Version says:

Thou shalt have no other Gods before me.

The question is, who do you think this "me" is? The churches have misinterpreted this meaning for thousands of years.

In Jeremiah 2:13, Mr. Lamsa's translation says:

For my people have...forsaken me, the fountain of living waters,

The King James Version says:

For my people have...forsaken me the fountain of living waters,

In Mr. Lamsa's translation, Spirit, or the entity called *me*, clearly defines itself as "the fountain of living waters." Notice the first comma is missing in King James, making the meaning unclear.

To understand Spirit as living waters and ourselves as made of Spirit is to understand the true meaning of the word "*me*." The difference between the God of religion and God as *me* is that I have to take 100 percent responsibility for my thinking, behavior, and wellness at all times. I have to know how I am *using* the Spirit Energy I am made of at each moment and endeavor to think highest-quality good thoughts at all times, in contrast to a belief in a religious God that I pray to, asking Him to forgive my sins and heal my body. With God as *me*, I have 100 percent control over my own health, wealth, and happiness. With the God of religion, I give responsibility for myself to circumstances and elements beyond my control and pray for deliverance.

Science has proved that we are made mostly of water,

but have you ever thought of yourself as water in the form of a body rather than as a body full of water? The difference between the water our body is made of and any other water is that the water in our body is infused with life. You know how easily water can change form. You just put it into a vessel of a different shape and its form automatically changes. But water can also change its appearance, texture, and structure from ice to liquid to vapor, so it is completely pliable and adaptable. Water will do anything you want it to do, and your body is made mostly of water. In fact, you are made of Living Waters as pure Spirit Energy.

The Inca understood that the Energy that powered their bodies *was* the immense force they called Great Spirit. They knew how to command the energy to shapeshift their bodies into eagles, falcons, and jaguars. The God of religion whom people pray to was unknown to them. Likewise, Jesus could transform Himself into invisible vapor in an instant, which He did to protect Himself from being stoned. When He wanted to shift the energy, He *sent* his word to do the job.

For us to learn how to consciously control the living water or Spirit we are made of, we study the triune mental process called the Holy Trinity, which teaches us how to turn water into form or how to re-form something negative. In the First Position, the water in this process is unformed and is invisible as vapor. In the Second Position, the water is invisible in the deep mind but visible on the surface or screen of the mind as liquid. In the Third Position of the Holy Trinity, the outcome, as ice, is visibly formed into the result as your health, wealth, or happiness, depending on the choices you made and the feelings you applied in the Second Position.

To demonstrate, in the First Position of the Trinity, we will use a bowl full of steam, or vaporized water infused with life, to represent the "I" or the "*me*" of the "I AM." It represents you as Living Spirit Energy with all potential. Other words that would fit in the First Position are *self, mind, being, light, life,* and *creator.*

In the Second Position, the steam or vapor in the bowl becomes liquid water, representing the "AM," or the moving part of the mental process. The breakers in the ocean simulate the ebb and flow of your thoughts in this position. The surface of the water represents your mental screen where you can see words and visions that have risen to the surface of your mind. Whatever you are actively mulling over or feeling in any given moment appears on that screen as words and visions where you can see them by looking inward. What choice will I make? How do I feel about that? This is where you want to reason correctly to make the right choice so the result in the Third Position will turn out well. Other words that work in the Second Position are *move, feel, think, ponder, vacillate,* and *choose.*

In the Third Position of the Trinity, colored marbles in the bottom of the bowl can represent formed beliefs or conclusions in your deep mind that have become visible either on your body or in your experience. The actual result depends on the exact words and feelings you combined and chose in the Second Position. In the Spirit realm, the Third Position is represented by formed ice. Other words that work in this position are *manifest, result, form, conclude,* and *body.*

There is a catalyst as a fourth element that must be present in your mind for the manifested result you desire to appear. This catalyst is your POSITIVE FEELING. Your feeling is the female element, and the female is the producer. To manifest what you want, your feeling must be in perfect alignment with what you say you want and feel in your heart. Words alone are powerful, but the female words, which are the feeling words like LOVE, cause Spirit Energy to move. Your negative beliefs and your self-doubt can prevent you from manifesting the positive result you would otherwise create if your feelings were positive.

Several years ago I was packing to move from Eugene, Oregon, to Santa Barbara, California. I had a lot of stuff to pack, and I began to think, "It's hard to move," which was my feeling about all the work that moving requires. As I continued to think that, it became harder to move my legs forward to walk normally. It felt like my legs were full of concrete, and I was having to drag them along behind me. Then I realized that I was thinking that it was "hard to move," so I began to say out loud, "It's easy to move." The stiffness gradually left my legs, so I was able to walk normally again. You may think that directing Spirit Energy is not that literal, but it is.

Another example where intense feelings were present occurred after the sudden death of my eighteen-year-old son Michael. My feeling was, "I can't stand it." I don't think I ever said that out loud, but Spirit Energy reads your feelings and is ever ready to give you whatever you're thinking. As the days went by after his death, I began to limp. Then I realized I was feeling that I could not stand the pain of losing him. Even with tears running down my cheeks, I began to say out loud, "I *can* stand it." Losing him hurt like hell, but I had to choose whether I wanted to be crippled because of the death of my son or if I was willing to think something positive anyway. As I continued to say "I *can* stand it," the pain in my foot went away, and I stopped limping.

Thinking is an exact science, and the words you think cause exact results on your body and in your life all the time. Research has shown that we run at least 1,300 words through our Self-talk every minute, so we must be mindful of what we are thinking and feeling constantly. You can work miracles by choosing consciously to think something in a positive way no matter what just happened, especially when your health or your body is expressing something negative. Remember, ***your*** thinking controls what happens to your body, and you always have control over your own thinking, but you have to exercise the control.

Your biggest challenge is to identify the exact negative feeling you need to reverse for healing. That negative feeling is most likely what has created your illness. You always know what has upset you and how you feel about that. Once you identify your negative feeling, think it in reverse to heal yourself. You may not always be willing to change your negative attitudes, but that is your choice.

To keep yourself in good health, think and speak in positives. For instance:

I AM MAKING GOOD PROGRESS.
I MOVE FORWARD EASILY.
I CAN STAND IT.
(These words affect your legs and feet.)

I AM WELL SUPPORTED.
I SUPPORT MY OWN CHOICES.
(Words of support affect your hipbones and your prosperity.)

I CAN BEND. I AM FLEXIBLE.
(These words affect your muscles and your neck.)

I FEEL PEACEFUL. I AM RELAXING.
(These words affect your nerves.)

I LOVE TO LIVE. I LOVE MY LIFE. I AM STRONG.
(These words affect your heart.)

I HAVE LOTS OF COURAGE.
(This reflects in your stomach and digestion.)

I FEEL INSPIRED. I AM SO LUCKY.
(These words support your lungs.)

I AM PATIENT.
(Patience affects your liver. The opposite of patience is anger and impatience, which are extremely harmful negative feelings that can affect any part of your body.)

No matter what happens to you in life, always hold to the perfection of your body. Never settle for less than perfection, and never decide that there's something permanently wrong with you. Your words and beliefs about your body inform ***your*** Spirit Energy, and your Energy will exactly match your beliefs in Third Position form, because you are made of Living Water or Spirit that wants to amiably comply with whatever you believe. Always remember the LAW OF PROPORTION:

WHATEVER YOU THINK 51 PERCENT OF THE TIME WILL MANIFEST.

If you want to work miracles, you need to work on loving your-Self first so you're starting right. You want to get "Self-Love" programmed into your mind so it's rolling constantly in your Second Position. Say to your-Self, "Mary/Charles, I love you." The more you can love and believe in your-Self as originating from the greatest power in existence, whatever you want to call it, the more you will be able to achieve. You are always free to think all the positive thoughts you want, so there is nothing ever hindering you. As you gain experience in moving Spirit Energy with your positive thinking, your self-confidence will grow, and your growing successes will spur you on to greater achievements. When you really understand what it means to be made of "Great Spirit" Energy, you will be overwhelmed with love, appreciation, and fascination for what you already are.

LOVING YOUR S.E.L.F. –

Scientifically Evolving Life Force

I CONSCIOUSLY RECOGNIZE MY-SELF (with a capital S).

I AM AN ENTITY WORTH LOVING.

I BELIEVE IN MY-SELF. (This is immensely powerful.)

I LOVE AND APPRECIATE MY-SELF.

I SEE PERFECTION IN MY-SELF AND IN OTHERS. (No fault-finding)

I LIVE IN PEACE WITH MY-SELF.

I HAVE FAITH IN THE CREATIVE POWER OF MY THOUGHT.

I CAN OVERCOME ANYTHING IF I CHANGE MY MIND.

I CAN CHANGE MY MIND. (I do it all the time.)

I HAVE DIVINE SELF-WORTH.

I AM A PRECIOUS TREASURE, A DIVINE BEING.

I HAVE INTEGRITY.

I LOVE MY-SELF AS A MAGNIFICENT BEING OF LIGHT.

I RESPECT MY-SELF.

I PRAISE MY-SELF FOR EVERY LITTLE THING.

I DESERVE THE BEST OF EVERYTHING LIFE HAS TO OFFER.

I REFUSE TO WORRY BECAUSE IT IMPROVES NOTHING.

I AM ENCIRCLED AND PROTECTED BY DIVINE WHITE LIGHT.

I LET MY LIGHT SO SHINE.

HEALING AFFIRMATIONS

MY THINKING CAUSES. EVERY DAY IN EVERY WAY MY LIFE GETS BETTER.

I TREAT MYSELF SWEET, KIND AND LOVING IN MY THOUGHTS, ACTIONS, AND DEEDS.

I AM CHANGING MY MIND FROM NEGATIVE TO POSITIVE ALL THE TIME.

I TREAT MYSELF LIKE THE DEAREST, MOST CHERISHED PERSON I WILL EVER KNOW.

I ADD POSITIVE WORDS TO MY MIND ON PURPOSE EVERY MINUTE EVERY DAY.

I AM BLESSED. I AM THE LUCKIEST PERSON IN THE WHOLE WORLD.

I THINK IN A POSITIVE WAY TO CREATE POSITIVE EXPERIENCES IN MY LIFE.

IF I WANT A QUALITY LIFE, I HAVE TO THINK QUALITY THOUGHTS, ESPECIALLY MY THOUGHTS ABOUT MYSELF.

I AM QUALITY OF THE HIGHEST CALIBER.

I AM MADE IN THE IMAGE AND LIKENESS OF THE CREATOR FROM THE VERY SAME CREATIVE SUBSTANCE. HE/SHE USED MORE OF HIM/HER-SELF TO MAKE ME.

I LOVE AND PRAISE MYSELF AS A DIVINE BEING, A HIGHLY VALUED CHILD OF GOD.

I AM GRATEFUL FOR EVERY GOOD THING IN MY LIFE.

MY BURDEN IS LIGHT ENERGY CONTROLLED BY MY FEELINGS AND ATTITUDES.

I USE MY SPIRIT ENERGY WISELY MOMENT BY MOMENT.

I KNOW WHO AND WHAT I AM–OMNISCIENT (infinite awareness), OMNIPOTENT (unlimited power), OMNIPRESENT (ubiquitous). EVERYTHING IS ENERGY.

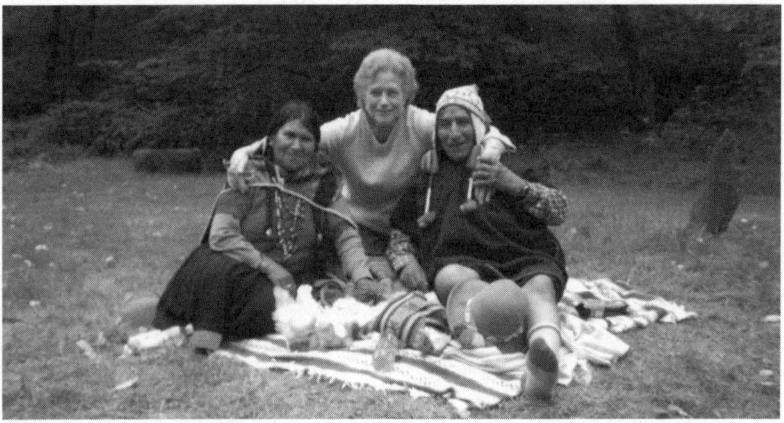

doña Bernadina, Nancy Harris, and don Humberto Soncco Quispe

CHAPTER FOUR

'ORGAN'-IZE YOUR ATTITUDES

THE MALE VIRTUES

Many centuries ago the Mayans closed their eyes and journeyed forward in time to foresee a specific period that some of us have now lived through: December 22-25, 2012. To journey forward in shamanic terminology is called a Destiny Retrieval. The Mayans predicted that our sun and other planetary bodies would align during this time. The Hopi elders who witnessed this event in 2012 verified that this planetary alignment did in fact take place. They could see it happen by looking inward into the dark mental space where their words form with their eyes closed. The National Aeronautics and Space Administration reported that there were no unusual planetary alignments at all. NASA expected to see this event by looking outward into space through their telescopes. If Edgar Cayce had failed to close his eyes and look inward to find the answers he needed to help his clients, there would be no books written about his work, and he would not now be known as "the sleeping prophet."

Learning to look inward to see what is going on in your mind and in your life is vital for each of us. So, to let you practice looking inward, we're going to take a journey.

You can put on a blindfold, or just dim the lights and close your eyes. To take a journey, you have to find the screen of your mind. You will know you are looking at it when you can see the stars in the night sky while you are looking inward. Sometimes it takes a minute or two to see the stars clearly, so be patient with the process. If you have trouble finding your mental screen when you look inward, you can try putting the palms of your hands tightly over your eyes in a very dark room. Then open your eyes, and you will see your mental screen reflecting on the palms of your hands as you look outward. Choose the way that works best for you, so here we go.

You are taking a journey to the Sahara Desert in northern Africa, and you've just arrived by van at your village destination. The Sahara is the largest hot desert in the world and the third largest desert after Antarctica and the Arctic. It's extremely hot here, but you are fairly comfortable in your hat, sunglasses, and loose clothing. As you begin to walk around, you see olive trees and a little vegetation growing here and there. You might see a cheetah, scorpions, or lizards, but the only domestic animals you see are camels and goats. Your long-time dream has been to have the experience of riding a camel, and now you see a man dressed in a long robe and a turban leading a camel straight toward you. The camel master commands the animal to kneel down right in front of you. Your dream is about to come true, so without hesitation you eagerly climb up into the saddle, and then the camel slowly stands up and begins to move forward. How does that feel? What do you see, and what happens? Go there now…

Now the ride is coming to an end. As the camel kneels down, you slide off, come back into the room, and open your eyes. Reflect for a moment on what happened.

To see yourself riding a camel, you were using your mental screen on the *face* or *surface* of your mind. It's important to learn to use this part of yourself successfully for conscious creating and intentional healing. You can use this screen to project positive words or reverse negative words to heal yourself of medically incurable illnesses, or to visualize new programs for positive future experiences.

I want to tell you a little more about my friend and client named Esther, whom I have mentioned previously. In addition to having problems with her sight, she also had diabetes, chronic constipation, and lymph problems. She lived, as most people do, by looking outward into the world of perception, and for her, "out there" was all that existed. So when I asked her to monitor her thinking and watch her attitudes, she could not find her thoughts to monitor. She had no conscious recognition of her Self as a being who thinks. All she was aware of was what she could see going on around her.

Esther was a woman who never threw anything away. The rooms in her home and garage were filled with piles of boxes full of unorganized things that she had collected over many years of living in her home. Even in the master bedroom you had to walk around piled-high boxes to get into the room. This disorganized clutter in her home was constricting the natural flow of energy in her body, causing constipation and messing up her blood chemistry.

The way you keep your home reflects the way you think, as organized or disorganized, living in the past or living in the now. Esther was dragging along all the old clutter and clothes from years gone by, and her body was in crisis, unable to release waste and poisons. One of the tables in her bedroom was completely covered with pill bottles, way too much medicine for one person to be taking. When I asked her about them she said she wasn't taking most of them anymore. She told me that when she got out of the shower, she would take off her shower cap and shake it three times while she said out loud, "Father, Son, and Holy Ghost." I asked her what she thought that would do for her. She said she didn't know, but she hoped it would do some good.

In the spiritual readings I did for her in an effort to save her sight, her spirit guides urgently pleaded with her, "Hurry up! Get rid of the old clutter." They said she was running out of time to help herself, but Esther flatly refused. She said, "No. I won't get rid of anything." She was set in her ways and flatly refused to cooperate. When she died several months later, she was completely blind. If you want your health to change, you have to be willing to change your negative attitudes and your negative behaviors.

One of the habits that Esther had was chronic fault-finding and the need to control her grown daughters. She loved and approved of one of her daughters, who lived with her husband on the East Coast. This daughter was attractive, and Esther could not say enough good things about her, and was very loving to her when she came to visit. The elder daughter was single, in her late thirties, a little heavy-set, and struggling to make a living as a choir director in Los Angeles. Esther would rant at this daughter over the telephone and was constantly finding fault with her. The last I heard about this daughter, she had been diagnosed with cancer and was really struggling to support herself and get well.

Fault-finding is now thought to be a dysfunctional illness, right along with drugs, alcohol, mental illness, sex addiction, and gambling. Dr. Daniel Amen, a noted psychiatrist, said on Oregon Public Broadcasting that the cause of the fault-finding attitude is the lack of a chemical called serotonin in the brain. This medical opinion implies the belief that our attitudes are controlled by chemicals in our blood chemistry. But, as an Energy Healer, I know that the exact opposite is true. Our positive and negative attitudes produce and regulate the chemicals in our bloodstream. Having the attitude of criticism and finding fault *causes* a lack of serotonin in the brain. Your attitudes are your own choice, which means you always have complete control over your own blood chemistry and over your health. If you don't like what you're getting, you have to be willing to correct yourself and think something positive. If Esther could have consciously reversed her attitude to loving herself and praising her daughter, rather than voicing all the criticism and fault-finding, serotonin could have reappeared naturally in her blood chemistry.

Doctors try to fix our chemical lack artificially with pills and drugs, but healing chronic illness without medicine always requires a reversal of your negative attitudes and behaviors. A person who becomes aware that his own negative attitudes are causing his chemical lack can re-supply it and heal himself by changing something in his life, his job, or his relationships, so his feelings and attitudes become positive and harmonious again. Trying to control and change other people is never the answer to healing yourself. Your positive attitudes will always reproduce the needed chemicals in your bloodstream naturally.

Diabetes is a major health problem in the world. A person with this illness may have tried so hard and for so long to control or correct someone else who is not cooperating that he feels distraught, exasperated, and that all sweetness is gone in that relationship or even in life. The pancreas is the organ in your body that reflects sweetness, so when you forget to be sweet, which is a virtue, it stops producing insulin, and you are diagnosed with diabetes. To get well, you have to give up the notion that you can change other people if you just keep trying, and concentrate instead on correcting your own negative attitudes, behaviors, and your need to control others. Choose to be sweet again, and allow other people to live their own lives in their own way.

YOUR THINKING CAUSES.
LOVING YOURSELF HEALS DYSFUNCTION.

Other negative attitudes that can **cause** chemical imbalances in your bloodstream and prevent your healing are:

1. HATING YOURSELF MORE THAN YOU LOVE YOURSELF, which causes dysfunction (alcoholism, drug addiction, and depression). If you've never really thought about that, begin to consciously say, "I love myself." It could save your life.
2. FINDING FAULT WITH OTHERS, which can create faults in your own body because you are the thinker. Find something good to say, or say nothing.
3. BELIEVING IN NEGATIVE IDEAS, like old age, conta-

gion, or choosing to stay sick to get more attention. The only things that can happen to your body are what you accept and allow.

4. BELIEVING TELEVISION COMMERCIALS THAT SELL SICKNESS. In January they sell the flu. Dr. Bernie Siegel said in an international on-line conference out of Singapore in November 2015, (which I was also invited to participate in), "Hundreds of thousands of people die every year because they are given (prescribed) the wrong medicine."
5. REFUSING TO FORGIVE, so you continue to entertain your negative feelings. Harboring a negative will never turn out positive.
6. CLAIMING THAT YOU *HAVE* THE ILLNESS. As long as you continue to claim it, you continue to re-create it. Begin to say, "I used to have it, but not now." Stop supporting what you don't want.
7. EXPECTING SOMEONE ELSE TO HEAL YOU. Your own positive feelings move the energy in the right direction. Physician, heal thyself.
8. FEELING GUILT OR REMORSE. Find a way to acquit yourself, because these feelings can cause serious pain in your body if continued.
9. DOUBTING YOURSELF. Your thoughts have God-Power. The more you believe in yourself, the more success you will have in every way.
10. ENTERTAINING FEAR AND ANGER CAN NEGATIVELY AFFECT ANY ORGAN IN YOUR BODY, so try not to entertain them. Remember that thinking the word PRAISE brings you security, which is protection

and money, and thinking the word PATIENCE helps you break your attitude of impatience, which is anger. So think these power words to combat fear and anger.

In one of my workshops, a class participant named Helen said she had been feeling hatred toward her husband, who had recently left her after being unfaithful. She said a friend told her that it was good to honor her negative feelings and just let them happen. But when feelings are involved, you have to choose what you're going to allow yourself to think. After the death of my son Michael, I was crying, limping, and feeling much sorrow, but I knew that if I continued to concentrate on those negative feelings, I would create more sorrow in my life, so I chose to think about something else. What we concentrate on most is what we create more of.

I said to Helen, "When you have to let go of someone you would rather hold onto, it hits you in the bowels." She replied, "I did have trouble with my bowels." The bowels reflect mercy and loving kindness (or lack of it) to one's self. The function of the bowels is to release, but when your feeling is that you would rather keep what you have to release in life (like your child), or when you would rather release what you have to keep, (like your job), this conflict in your feelings can result in angry bowel syndrome or Crohn's disease. No matter what just happened, you have to allow the process of life to unfold as it will, and deal with it in a positive, congenial, flexible way without trying to run the world yourself.

When you're going through a difficult time and feeling heavy negative emotions, choose to HOLD high-level positive words in your mind to counteract your negative feelings until they pass. Flashing and holding these positive power words on your mental screen will create positive resistance to the negative feelings that are trying to ruin your good health. Some power words to hold in your mind are:

GRATITUDE, SERENITY, COMFORT, HOPE, MERCY, COURAGE, STRENGTH, BLISS

Jesus understood that everything is energy, and He knew how to *use* the energy to heal, to become invisible, and to manifest whatever He wanted instantly. When He healed people, even long-distance, He *sent his word* to heal them. I used to wonder, "What word did He send?" but Scripture does not say. Of course, the answer to that question is that He could read their mind, so He sent them the direct opposite positive-feeling word to reverse the negative-feeling word they had thought that created their illness. The positive word He sent canceled out their negative energy, and they were instantly healed. We can learn to do this too. Jesus said, "I and the Father are One," meaning: *We are what God is, Living Energy.*

You've heard people ask, "Why does God allow wars and all these awful things that happen?" To ask that question shows a misconception of what God is.

WE ARE MADE OF THE GOD ENERGY.

OUR THINKING controls the quantum field of Living Energy that IS GOD. In Him (or *AS Him, Her, or It*) we live, move, and have our being. Our thinking, feelings, attitudes, and choices cause this God Energy to move and to create whatever we feel most deeply about. The most important questions to ask yourself every moment are "How am I using my God Energy right now? Have I remembered to love myself today? What am I creating with my words and thoughts? Are they positive or negative?" Be SELF-AWARE! Quantum physics verifies that everything is vibrating energy that is pushed in the direction of your thoughts.

The Inca understood that everything is pure energy, and they called this powerful force "Great Spirit." The word *spirit* means "breath or life force" and also "attitude, disposition, feeling, or frame of mind." You, as pure Spirit Energy, are composed of earth, water, air, fire, and the prana (or spirit) that breathes life into these elements. These are all components of the Medicine Wheel, a symbol found in many cultures all over the globe, representing healing in a shamanic sense, as well as a way to gain access to the essence of existence.

Dr. Masaru Emoto says in his book, *The Hidden Messages in Water,* that your body is mostly water, with about ninety chemical elements. He found that *every attitude* you have produces a particular chemical in your bloodstream. Feeling *anger* produces lead, *despair* produces steel, *irritation* produces mercury, *sadness* produces aluminum, and *stress* produces zinc. Dr. Emoto found that when you think *love* and *gratitude* you become a beautiful shining crystal of light filled with purified blood and water.

THE MALE VIRTUES:

To understand the correlation between the words you think and the organs in your body, we will now study the seven major Virtues that represent mental or spiritual *organ*-ization. The word *virtue* means "Moral excellence, uprightness of conduct" and "conformity to a standard of right as divine law or the highest good." Here we will discuss the three male virtues, the Heart, Stomach, and Lungs, represented by animals with claws. The four female virtues, the Blood, Liver, Kidneys, and Brain, are represented by animals with hooves and will be discussed later.

If you think of your body as an *organ*-ized system controlled by the virtues, healing yourself from medically incurable illness becomes possible. Particular virtuous words relating to certain morals govern the health of each organ in your body. To maintain your health consciously, you have to know the positive words that represent each organ, so you can consciously think these words to heal yourself if you find any particular organ malfunctioning.

The animals that relate to the male virtues are the Bear, representing the Heart; the Lion, representing the Stomach; and the Fox, representing the Lungs. These animals relate to the text from Isa. 11:6-9:

The wolf shall dwell with the lamb,
and the leopard shall lie down with the kid;
and the calf and the young lion and the fatling together;
and a little child shall lead them.

If you Google the painting called "Peace" by William Strutt, you may be able to find a copy of this painting that shows the animals in this Scripture.

THE HEART, represented by the Bear, is the first male Virtue we will study. The function of the heart, or cardiac muscle, is to pump blood out into the arteries and circulate it throughout the body, delivering food and oxygen from the lungs to the organs and tissues. The blood returns to the heart through the veins. It is then pumped into the lungs to replace the oxygen, and then back into the heart to recycle again.

The positive-feeling words, virtues or morals that control and regulate the HEART:

Strength, Power, Self-Reliance, Virility, Usefulness, Living In The Now, The Ability To Bear

The opposite negative-feeling words or misuse of the virtue:

Death, Weakness, Infirmity, Disability, Impotency, Uselessness, Memories, Burdens

When a parent has many children to support and has worked many years at a difficult job with little rest, he or she may feel that his or her burdens are too hard to bear any longer. This attitude causes *arteriosclerosis*, in which "the walls of small arteries become thickened due to aging or hypertension, inhibiting or blocking the flow of blood from the heart." To recover, that person would need to release his burden and change his lifestyle. My former husband, Ray, had that problem. He was a good father who believed in taking care of his family. For years he worked as a purchasing agent, and I taught piano at home. He got along well as long as we had three children to support, but when our fourth child came along, Ray began to have some pain around his heart, which he did finally overcome.

THE STOMACH, represented by the Lion, is another male Virtue. The function of the stomach, as part of the digestive system, is to break down food into substances that can be absorbed and used by the body for energy, growth, and repair. Food travels down the esophagus and into the stomach, where mucus, hydrochloric acid, and the enzyme pepsin break it down into peptones. The chemicals, together with the churning action of the stomach muscles, reduce the food to a semi-liquid that passes into the small intestine.

Virtues, morals, or positive-feeling words that control and regulate the STOMACH:

Courage, Reason, Heroism, Boldness, Competence, Appetite, Pleasure

The opposite negative-feeling words or misuse of the virtue:

Cowardice, Disgust, Repulsion, Inadequate, Absurdity, Timidity, Discomfort

Many years ago I had a beautiful young blond neighbor named Sheila. She was married to a policeman named Paul who worked on the narcotics squad in San Jose, California. They had an eighteen-month-old child named Betty. In the course of Paul's police work he met someone that he had an affair with. When Sheila found out, she became sick to her stomach and began heaving. Her child also had an upset stomach and diarrhea as a sympathetic reflection of her mother's feelings of disgust.

THE LUNGS are the third male Virtue we will study, and are represented by the Fox. We use our lungs to inhale oxygen from the air and to exhale carbon dioxide to sustain life. We breathe about twelve times a minute, and about 282 cubic feet of air in twenty-four hours.

Virtues, morals, or positive-feeling words that control and regulate the LUNGS:

Hope, Inspiration, Enjoyment, Encouragement, Optimism, Wisdom, Confidence, Enthusiasm, Security, Feeling Lucky, Happiness

The opposite negative-feeling words or misuse of virtue:

Despair, Listless, Sorrow, Discouraged, Foolish, Pessimistic, Despondent, Indifferent, Depressed

When I was working toward my Master's Degree in music, midterms were approaching, and I had a lot of studying to do. I sat down at the table and opened my books. But I really didn't want to be sitting there doing that. I just wasn't in the mood. As I started to read, my nose began to run. Soon I felt like I must be catching a cold. Then I realized what I was thinking. I was not enjoying what I was doing, so I had a little talk with myself.

"Who decided to enroll in school to get this degree?" "I did." And who cares about making good grades?" "I do." "Well, then what is your problem?" And in that moment, as I observed my negative attitudes and changed my mind, my nose dried up quickly. Next time you feel like you're catching a cold, ask yourself what you're not enjoying. Either start enjoying it or stop doing it. Do not blame it on contagion. That's just a belief!

In conclusion, always choose to support what is GOOD. Hold to the perfection of your body no matter what happens, and always believe in yourself. Your God-Energy is yours to control. Your attitudes create your health.

CHAPTER FIVE

FINE-TUNE YOUR FEELINGS

THE FEMALE VIRTUES

In the beginning God created the heaven and the earth.

Gen. 1:1

For this to happen, God, as a conscious presence, had to be aware of itself. Waking up to your Self is the quintessential goal for each of us.

And the earth was without form and void;
and darkness was upon the face of the deep.
And the Spirit of God moved
upon the face of the waters.

Gen. 1:2

The *deep* symbolizes "water or deep mind." A *spirit* is an "attitude or feeling" (like the spirit of Christmas). We have lots of attitudes; some are good and some are not so good. This Scripture tells us that when our attitudes move on the *face* of the mind, it causes something else to move. The *face* is the *screen* or *surface* on top of the deeper part of the mind. *Water* symbolizes unformed thought-in-solution as potential. Your feelings and beliefs (as Spirit Energy) cause the waters (as thoughts) to move (toward a manifested result).

And God said, 'Let there be light,' and there was light.

Gen. 1:3

As you know, our light comes from the sun. Why did God need to create light? In darkness there is no light of understanding. When we shed a little light on something, we begin to understand that our own thoughts move Spirit Energy, and light makes vision possible. Why create something that cannot be seen? Light also signifies the attitude of love that warms our feelings, as opposed to the darkness of hatred that chills and kills.

And God saw the light, that it was good.

Gen. 1:4

The renowned physicist David Bohm said, "All matter is frozen light." By "frozen" he refers not to temperature but to *seeming* solidity. We are literally made of light, and light is pure energy vibrating at various frequencies. We are made of what God is, energy that travels about 186,281 miles per second. How fast can you shift your thought from here to the moon? And there you are! Jesus said, "My burden is Light."

Dr. Jacob Liberman says in his book, *Light Medicine of the Future,* "The human body is truly a living photocell that is energized by the sun's light. Since light is recognized as having a profound effect on all living things, and since our perception of light is by way of our eyes, it becomes evident that the function of the eyes may not be for *seeing* alone."

Albert Szent-Gyorgyi, Nobel Prize winner and the discoverer of vitamin C, said, "All the energy we take into our body is derived from the sun." He saw that through the process of photosynthesis the sun's energy is stored in plants, so when we eat our vegetables we are literally eating light. Our digestive organs break down, transfer, store, and utilize this light as living energy.

The Inca worshipped the sun and used sunlight for healing. They knew that by concentrating on what they wanted, the Creative Energy would move to conform to their thinking, so they consciously dreamed their world into being. They could shape-shift their own bodies into other living creatures and back again into so-called human form, because they understood that light, as energy, could be molded into any shape they wanted it to be.

And God said, 'Let us make man in our image,
after our likeness, and let them have dominion…
over all the earth.'

Gen. 1:26

Webster defines *our* as "belonging to us, or to ourselves as possessors."

So God created man in his own image,
male and female created he them.

Gen. 1:27

God was our progenitor, forefather, and patternmaker. His name was I AM, and when I say His name followed by any other word, I AM HAPPY, or I AM SAD, my energy moves in that direction because I AM MADE OF GOD'S ENERGY, and the Spirit of my words moves the energy I am made of.

Created in God's image, we too can beget and reproduce male and female offspring. Just like God, as we think, so we are. As long as we think joyful, peaceful, harmonious thoughts, and believe in ourselves, we keep our body full of Light Energy and good health. But we are learning that when we become emotional and our *feelings* are mostly negative, then dark energy and illness can result. So the way to heal yourself of any illness and work your miracle is to *reverse* your negative feelings back to positive feelings as fast as you can. When you shift the balance of your energy back to positive, the result will be automatic wellness. To be reborn out of the so-called physical world of humankind into the world of the Spirit, think of your *Self* always and only as Light Energy.

Like our Creator, we have infinite abilities, infinite choices, and infinite potential, in spite of any beliefs to the contrary we have about ourselves. This would have to be true for us to have the energy to live forever, moving from one body to the next in our soul's journey through many lifetimes. When we die in each lifetime, our eighth chakra begins to create a new body temple for our infinite Light Energy body to indwell as we travel onward.

THE FEMALE VIRTUES:

Specifically, the word *virtue* means, "merit, value, worth, chastity, and purity." It also means:

- Conformity to a standard of right, as Divine Law or the highest good
- Moral excellence
- Integrity of character

- Uprightness of conduct
- Exertion of your abilities in doing good
- Wisdom based on knowledge that makes you act in accordance with the good

The health of each organ or system in your body is controlled by specific virtuous words. When an organ or part of your body begins to hurt or malfunction, it's because of a particular negative feeling, attitude, or emotion that you have mentally entertained. If you know which positive words or feelings govern each organ, you can correct your mistake in thought and relieve your pain by thinking these positive controlling words consciously and consistently to overcome your negative feelings. By doing this, you will reverse your energy from negative to positive, automatically rebalance your blood chemistry, and heal your illness. What you're going to think becomes your choice. Rather than allowing negative words or feelings that make you sick to take you down, you consciously choose to think positive words to overturn your negative feelings and keep you well.

Each organ or system in your body has a corresponding ànimal that characterizes the traits of that virtue. We have already studied the organs that represent the Male Virtues. They are the heart, lungs, and stomach, represented by animals with claws–the bear, fox, and lion. Now we will study the organs that represent the Female Virtues. They are the liver, kidneys, and blood, represented by animals with hooves–the cow, lamb, and llama. By studying the Virtues, you will know the positive words to think to heal an illness affecting the organs they represent.

If you will Google the famous painting called "Peace"

by William Strutt, you will see pictures of the animals that represent the organs. The brain is represented by the picture of the Little Child. The Angel represents a high level of Christ consciousness, including your merit, value, chastity, purity, and excellence.

THE LIVER - COW

The Liver is part of the digestive system. It's the largest organ in the body, weighing three to four pounds. The liver handles the basic substances your body runs on–proteins, carbohydrates, and fats. Because we eat proteins in various forms, the liver has to synthesize the raw proteins from the blood with its enzymes. It also extracts and neutralizes poisons and wastes, and then creates proteins acceptable to our body.

Virtues, morals, or positive-feeling words that control and regulate the LIVER:

> **Patience, Contentment, Satisfaction, Calm, Composed, Relaxed, Untiring Industry In Doing, Forebearing Hardship Or Difficulty Without Moral Change, Cheerfully Uncomplaining Under Any And All Circumstances**

The opposite negative-feeling words or misuse of the virtue:

> **Irritable, Complaining, Nagging, Quick-tempered, Tense, Restless, Unstable, Vacillating, Impetuous, Uneasy**

THE KIDNEYS - LAMB

The kidneys are part of the excretory system. Their function is to remove urea from the blood and waste products resulting from chemical processes within the body that enable it to grow, survive, and reproduce. The kidneys are situated at the back of the abdomen, below the diaphragm, one on each side of the spine. They filter the blood and then re-absorb water and other substances back into the blood. The waste product flows into the ureter, which leads to the bladder.

Virtues, morals, or positive-feeling words that control and regulate the KIDNEYS:

> **Innocence, Purity, Truth, Gentle, Mild, Refined, Kind, Peaceful, Tender, Merciful, Without Blame Or Guilt, Easily Subdued, Clean, Simple, Trusting, Soft**

The opposite negative-feeling words or misuse of the virtue:

> **Feeling Guilty, Impure, Telling Lies, Easily Misled Or Fooled, Vulnerable To Being Cheated, Naïve, No Self-Defense**

This is the story of my friend Lucille (the grandmother), Rhonda (her daughter), and Amanda (her granddaughter). Many years ago Lucille called me one evening. Her doctor had diagnosed her with cryptogenic cirrhosis of the liver. Lucille was in her sixties, and she knew I was a spiritual healer. She had told me previously that her grown daughter Rhonda had been born with an imperfectly functioning kidney. After surgery, the baby was left with one good kidney. Lucille was still seeking answers as to why this problem had occurred.

I told her that the kidneys represent innocence, purity, and truth, so malfunction of a kidney may indicate that a lie has been told. She was silent on the phone for a moment, and then she said, "I lied to my family and tried to make them believe that my husband was the baby's father." As a young woman Lucille had been a beauty, and she revealed to me that she had been involved in an extramarital affair. She and her husband had divorced because of it, leaving her with lots of grief, anger, and guilt. As the years went by, her unhealed emotions reflected on her body as a diseased liver. Lucille listened quietly as I explained that she had misused the virtue of Truth by telling a big lie, which reflected on her baby's kidney, causing it to malfunction and to be lost through surgery in infancy.

You can never fool yourself. You always know what you did, or said, or thought. The negative result of some virtue *you* misused can manifest on the most vulnerable member of your family–your child or even your pet–rather than on you. A lie can also become what the Bible calls "Sins of the Father" and create kidney (or other) problems for your descendants through seven generations, unless the karmic imprint of that lie is removed through a shamanic soul retrieval.

Many years after Lucille's death, Rhonda's grown married daughter Amanda, now in her thirties, was also having kidney problems. She had worked with doctors for ten years, and they could not heal her. I suspected she might be having Sins of the Father karmic problems because of her grandmother's lie. However, in giving Amanda an energy treatment and a spiritual reading to investigate the cause, I found that it was not a karmic problem. Amanda's kidney problems were being caused by poor choices she was making. She was choosing to use substances that were creating impurities in her kidneys and in her blood. I gave her two energy treatments (a Soul Retrieval and a Seven Chakra Illumination), after which her doctor said her kidneys were in remission. I find it interesting that Webster's Dictionary says the word *remission* means "the act of pardoning sin or offense," and the word *forgiveness* is a synonym.

THE BLOOD - LLAMA

The blood is part of the cardiovascular system, which includes the blood vessels and the heart. Its function is to carry oxygen, hormones, food molecules, and other substances throughout the body.

Virtues, morals, or positive-feeling words that control and regulate the BLOOD:

Love For Self And Others, Persistence,
Endurance, Tolerance, Consistence,
To Cherish, Abide, Support, Yield, Sustain

The opposite negative-feeling words or misuse of the virtue:

Undue Sense Of Responsibility, Obligation,
Too Serious, Grave, Gloomy, Feeling Heavy,
Hateful, Driven, Suffering, Easily Imposed On

Many years ago before I became an energy healer, an attractive young woman named Katy and her ten-year-old daughter Melanie began taking piano lessons from me, and we became good friends. I had watched Katy and her handsome husband, Jim, at the fairgrounds during a sportsmen's show, casting fishing line in an effort to drive sales for their local sporting goods store. One day Katy came to her piano lesson and told me that she had been diagnosed with leukemia. Leukemia is a malignant disease in which the bone marrow and other blood-forming organs produce abnormal white blood cells called leukocytes. They suppress the production of normal white cells, red cells, and platelets, which leads to infection, anemia, bleeding, and enlargement of certain organs.

Katy said she was having a lot of marital problems and that her husband was cheating on her. After several months of illness with no improvement, Katy decided to fly to Texas to have a blood transfusion. That was the last time I ever saw her. She never recovered from the procedure.

Our bones are governed by the virtuous word HARMONY. Too much of the opposite negative word, DISHARMONY, can lead to broken bones and malignant diseases such as leukemia. Thinking love and harmony more than you think the opposite negative words will keep your blood and your bones healthy. Remember, whatever you think 51 percent of the time is what will reflect on your body or in your life.

You have to stop believing that you have no control over your own blood chemistry. If you want healthy blood, you have to think the virtuous health-giving words that sustain it most of the time. Thinking SELF-LOVE is at the top of the list. You want LOVE FOR YOURSELF AS A DIVINE BEING flowing around in your blood and nourishing every part of your body every moment of the day.

Never stop thinking SELF-LOVE. It will help you through any situation.

THE BRAIN - LITTLE CHILD

There are three different regions in the brain: the hindbrain, the midbrain, and the forebrain. The hindbrain, which includes the cerebellum, is concerned mainly with motor activities and body movements. The brain stem in the midbrain links the brain with the spinal cord. The brain stem controls heart rate, blood pressure, swallowing, coughing, breathing, and unconsciousness. The cerebrum is located in the forebrain. It handles thought, memory, consciousness, and higher mental processes like decision-making. The cerebrum also coordinates muscle activity, facial expressions, and positioning of limbs before standing or walking. The hypothalamus lies at the base of the brain. It controls eating, sleeping, and temperature control, and connects with areas involved with our senses, behavior, and memory.

Virtues, morals, or positive feeling words that control and regulate the BRAIN:

Understanding–Especially For Your-Self,
All The Virtues Combined

You are the Creator as a multi-dimensional being controlling waves of Light Energy with your every thought. To preserve your body in a state of health, your goal is to think good virtuous words every moment across the board, especially the words you use to think about your-Self.

Every organ in your body has virtuous words controlling it. Now that you have learned the virtuous words that govern the major organs, we will have a little quiz. You can either write down your answers or just say them out loud. We'll begin with the Female Virtues, then shift to the Male Virtues. First, I will say a virtuous word. You name the organ that this word controls.

1. INNOCENCE
2. LOVE
3. PATIENCE
4. STRONG
5. INSPIRATION
6. COWARD

Now I will name a feeling. Say or write the organ it affects and the virtuous word to think to re-balance your energy.

7. I AM SO ANGRY.
8. I'M AFRAID TO DO THIS. MY BUTTERFLIES ARE ACTING UP.
9. I FEEL HOPELESS, DISCOURAGED, UNINSPIRED.
10. I FEEL SO MUCH DISHARMONY!

Answers for Quiz:
1) Kidneys 2) Blood 3) Liver 4) Heart 5) Lungs 6) Stomach 7) Liver - patience, contentment, satisfaction 8) Stomach - courage 9) Lungs - joy, hope, inspiration 10) Bones - harmony

Remember that anger and fear can cause problems anywhere in your body. Anger can express as inflammation, and fear can express as infection. Feeling anger at yourself is very unwise, no matter what has happened. Anger can cause you to do and say unreasonable things that may be hard to undo later. Reacting with anger or irritation can cause Crohn's disease in the bowels. Many people who have this problem have their intestines resectioned to make the pain go away. However, unless they also *cut out* their attitude of anger, they may find Crohn's disease just moves into the remaining sections of the intestines. If you choose to cut away the diseased organ without correcting your negative attitude, you may live to regret it, if you can live without your organs. Some people trust that their body will be better for having surgery, but this is not always true. I have heard people say after surgery, "I wish I'd never done that." Your organs are precious, and attitudes can be changed. Choose to practice and think the word *patience* the next time you catch yourself getting angry. You may save your organs and preserve your life.

It's important to be sensitive to the way you react to the events in your day, especially the events that aren't quite the way you want them to be. Analyze your reactions on the spot. Be SELF-AWARE. How did I just react? Was that *annoyance*, *irritation*, or *aggravation*? There are so many different forms of anger! How did I use my energy? Was I *critical*? Did I *find fault*? What was that feeling? Try to be as exact as possible. These negative feelings may be habitual, and if they reach 51 percent of your thinking on that subject, they will shift your energy and cause illness in your body.

Once you begin to catch yourself reacting in a negative way, you can begin to reverse that habit or pattern by saying to yourself, "I see what I just did. I reacted with aggravation. No! I will no longer react that way. Now I choose to react with patience, mercy, and loving kindness." As you begin to practice catching your own negative reactions and reversing them instantly, you will become better at it as you go along. You must have infinite patience to LET things happen in a natural manner.

In addition to monitoring your reactions, it's also important to keep your feelings in balance - not just negative to positive, but also "too much" or "too little" of a feeling. *Too much* can become "excessive or overly," and *too little* can become "deprivation or lack of." Either way, it's a negative. Middle of the road, or moderation, in all things concerning attitudes or feelings is best if you want to stay in a state of good health.

Allowing things to happen in a natural manner without trying to control other people is important for the sake of your own health. That also includes your grown married children. I know people who have made themselves very sick (often with diabetes), who just cannot stop trying to control what they see happening in someone else's life, but they fail to notice their own dysfunction at all. They know they don't feel well, and they may even take pills or shots daily just to stay alive, but they go right on trying to control others. They just don't like what the other person is doing. These people always mean to be helpful, but your illness always tells you that YOU are the person who needs to change.

William Walter said, "The person who gets sick is the person who is wrong." I used to wonder what he meant by that. The person who gets sick is the person who is thinking in negatives and finding the most fault. Positive thinking will always keep you well. St. Paul said, "Work out *your own* salvation." An illness is there to tell you that you are not doing something in the right way. We all learn from our mistakes. Learn to butt out of other people's business. And, "yes," your grown children qualify as "other people."

In spiritual healing, there is no quick fix. There is no magic pill. When you change your attitudes from negative to positive, your healing is automatic. You can work your own miracles at any time by being positive and loving to yourself and to others. You have to learn to think in reverse. Your body will always tell you which way you felt and reacted without fail.

King Solomon said, "With all thy getting, get wisdom. Get understanding." Pay attention to yourself and from now on start choosing consciously-controlled reactions rather than allowing old habitual emotional ones to control you any longer. There are always bad habits to break and good new ones to form. Your energy will produce for you either way you think it.

CHAPTER SIX

REVERSE YOUR FEELING – GET YOUR HEALING

My friend Gwen had just sold her home in Eugene, Oregon, and wanted to move to a location in Washington State, just south of the Canadian border. She had gone to that area to look for a home to buy, but she didn't know exactly where she wanted to be, so she found a home to rent in that general area. Then she asked me to do a spiritual reading to see where she was supposed to look for her new home, so I performed a Destiny Retrieval, which is a reading to foresee the future. What I saw was a rooster. It looked like a weather vane, and it was turning this way and that as if to say, "Look farther, look wider, and expand your search." So, she moved from Eugene into the house she had rented in northern Washington and went into the local police station to get licenses for her three big Labrador Retrievers.

At the police station she met her new neighbor, who worked there as a receptionist. While they were talking, a lady came in to ask the police to watch her house while she went away for the winter. She said to the receptionist, "Do you know of anyone who would like to buy a house?" The neighbor said, "Yes! *She* would," pointing to Gwen. The lady invited Gwen to follow her home, and there was the weather vane in the shape of a rooster on top of this lady's house. There was even a perfect yard for her dogs. Gwen bought the house and the rooster. This story is an example of someone who wanted to make a big change. She knew what she wanted, but she didn't know exactly where it was. Spirit opened the path directly to her goal, and she was led right to it.

Recently I said to Gwen, "When you put your desire into Spirit Energy, sooner or later you will connect with your goal." She replied, "All in God's good time!" God's good time is when your heart's feeling (which is your female element) and your knowing or reason (which is your male element) are in perfect agreement. As long as your mind or reason argue with your heart's desire, what you want will probably not appear. But when your heart and your mind work together and both say "Yes!" so the negative resistance is completely gone, that's when the energy shifts and the miracle happens. That is God's good time–union of the male and female elements (your knowing and your feeling) in perfect harmony. God's "good time" is also called *conception.*

YOUR EXPERIENCE IS EXACT TO YOUR PATTERNS OF THOUGHT

To demonstrate the exact way our mental patterns attract whatever we're experiencing, Dr. Alberto Villoldo uses the analogy of iron filings on a piece of glass being controlled and arranged by a magnet on the opposite side of the glass. Our habitual ways of thinking and reacting create our mental patterns. As you practice monitoring your thinking and begin to notice your own negative ways of reacting, you can begin to change and improve your habits and mental patterns consciously so your experiences will begin to improve. To shift energy, you have to know how to reverse what is being pulled or magnetized into your experience by thinking in the exactly opposite way. To reverse a negative experience, change your negative feelings to positive feelings on purpose. You will always know when your positive feelings are beginning to replace the negative words you have thought in the past, because good feelings come along naturally with the good words as you think them.

THINKING THE OPPOSITE FEELING WORDS PRODUCES THE OPPOSITE RESULT

In his book, *Awakened Imagination*, DeVorss Publications, Neville says, "Imagine yourself actually experiencing whatever you want from the *feelings* of your wish fulfilled, and you will grant to yourself what sleeping men ask of God." This means if you can imagine that you already have what you want to the point where you can *feel* how it would feel, you will shift your energy and consciously create what you want. When you manifest something you really want in your life, it will *feel* like a dream come true. It fills you with pleasure, joy, happiness, and great satisfaction, which makes you feel it all the more.

YOUR *FEELING* IS THE MOVER THAT SHIFTS THE ENERGY

Think of something that you would just love to have in your life. What is your dream or your heart's desire? Either write it down to clearly define it, or say it out loud. Now imagine that your dream just came true, and in this moment right now you are experiencing for the very first time how it feels to finally have it. Notice the words that come up in your mind. Are you thrilled? Do you love it? Is it comfortable to have it? Does it feel right? What needs to change if it doesn't feel right? Always pay attention to your feelings.

TO MANIFEST YOUR DREAM STOP SUPPORTING THE NEGATIVE FEELINGS THAT PREVENT IT

To maintain your body in good health and have peace in your life, you must learn to monitor and control your feelings, because they move the Creative Energy that you're made of in one direction or another. When disease or malfunction manifest on your body, it's always *your own negative feelings* that created it. Consciously reverse your feelings to the *exact opposite positive feelings* intentionally, and the Creative Energy will follow your thoughts exactly to heal you. Your balance or imbalance of positive-to-negative thinking always controls your health.

YOUR *FEELINGS* CONTROL AND REGULATE THE CHEMICALS IN YOUR BLOODSTREAM

Health is a choice. You can stubbornly go on with your negative feelings and stay sick, or practice Self-correction and get well. If only you could realize how infinitely powerful you are, you would endeavor to think high-level positive words all the time to use your Creative Energy wisely and correctly. The benefits to your health, wealth, and life would be immense.

In October 2011, Ray, my former husband of thirty-six years, passed away. Even though we had been divorced for sixteen years, I never stopped loving him. I just chose not to live with his drinking any more. I thought I was getting along pretty well with his passing until some of his belongings came into my possession. Then I began to remember how it used to be when we were happy, and all the memories came rushing back. I began to feel depressed, and my left foot and leg started hurting. As the days went by, I noticed that my legs didn't want to move forward when I walked, so I said out loud to my energy, "I move forward easily." After I said that a couple of times, what I saw rise up in my mind was "I can't move forward at all." By thinking these positive words out loud to reverse the energy, I was dumping the negative feelings in my mind that I had been entertaining. Apparently I felt that with Ray gone I could no longer move forward in my own life, so my legs were giving me exactly what I was feeling. If I allowed myself to become depressed and sorrowful over his death, it awakened old pains in my body that I thought I had overcome. So I found I had to lift my thoughts back up into a higher state of *peace, harmony, joy,* and *acceptance* to get out of pain again. As I became happier and more positive in my feelings, the pain in my legs disappeared.

Creative Energy, or Spirit, is potent power ever ready to be moved by your feelings and not to be taken lightly or misunderstood. You don't always consciously know what your feelings are, but the Creative Energy that your body is made of always knows what you're thinking the most and reflects that exact feeling perfectly on your body. If you pay attention to what your body is telling you about your feelings, you can learn a lot about yourself and about the way you think.

Spiritual healing is always about Self-correction. If your negative beliefs, opinions, and words do not change in your mind, the health of your body will not change either. You are the one who has to think the positive words to make your energy shift. No one else can do this for you.

Here are some words that denote negative feelings. If you were feeling this way, what positive word would you have to hold in your mind to reverse it to a positive feeling?

1) LACK 2) WORTHLESS 3) GRIEF 4) SELF-HATRED 5) ANGER 6) PAIN

Answers:

1) plenty, abundance 2) magnificent, supreme 3) joy, happiness 4) self-love 5) patience, self-control 6) great comfort

To heal my nine-year-old son Michael of congenital glaucoma, I had to say "*NO*" to my domineering mother-in-law and stand my ground. I had always said "*YES*" to her demands before. Michael's glaucoma vanished because I *reversed* my way of dealing with her. Rather than letting her push me around any longer, I pushed back. The doctors had said there was no medical cure for glaucoma, but I found there was a spiritual way to heal it by reversing the word "yes" to the word "no." I had to stop *feeling* that I needed to please other people and choose to honor my own feelings by pleasing myself for a change.

To heal myself when my left hipbone disconnected

from my spine after my son Jeff hanged himself, I reversed my feelings of separation from my son by saying, "Nothing can separate me," (meaning "I am connected") in spite of what Jeff chose to do. With that change of mind, the bones in my hip and spine reconnected perfectly and automatically. By consciously reversing your feelings, you can work the miracle of perfect healing on your own body. Always be aware of the things that upset you so will know what feelings to reverse.

How hard is it to reverse a word? Actually, it's *easy*. Is that a choice? *Yes*. For healing, can you think the positive word one time and reverse the energy? No, probably not if you've had the problem for a while. You have to hold the opposite positive word(s) in your mind until your thinking becomes 51 percent positive for your energy to shift. Remember, the positive word has to be the exact opposite of the negative feeling you entertained that made you sick.

If you have chosen a particular positive word to think to treat yourself and your illness still continues with no sign of letup, go back to the dictionary or thesaurus and choose a more precise word. Be scientific in your approach. The word that will shift the energy must embody the *exact opposite positive feeling* from the negative feelings you entertained that created your illness. In a thesaurus, the word *jealousy* may show nine antonyms (opposites). Maybe only one of those antonyms is the right one to reverse the illness you're working on. If you persist in treating yourself as correctly as you possibly can and your energy still does not shift, you may be dealing with other problems, such as karma, a curse, or a negative soul contract with Spirit. These can all be released through an energy treatment called a Soul Retrieval. The one thing that can absolutely prevent your healing is your own Self Doubt. The power of your own thought to heal you is, *without doubt,* the most omnipotent force in existence.

BELIEVE IN YOURSELF WITH ALL YOUR HEART, SOUL, AND MIND

When I was thirty-four years old, I had a bad case of pneumonia. I lived just south of Seattle, Washington, and it was January and very cold outside. My husband listened to me coughing and choking and saw me lying in bed for several days, not appearing to be improving at all. He called the doctor, bundled me up, and drove me through deep snow up the hill to the medical facility in Federal Way, Washington. I remember lying there on the doctor's table feeling that now I would be able to get well because I had seen the doctor. And sure enough, from that moment on I began to recover. I'm sure I took whatever medicine he prescribed over the next few days, but I knew it was my change of mind that healed me. I believed I was getting well.

I know now that pneumonia is the result of feeling *hopeless.* Shortly before I came down with pneumonia, I had been upset because my younger sister, Brenda, had died suddenly at age twenty-nine, and I was afraid her ex-husband, Bob, would inherit our grandfather's money. Bob was a drug addict, and Brenda was quite afraid of him. I had worried and fretted and felt hopeless over that scenario ever turning out as Grandfather would have wanted it to. Of course, as time went on it did turn out right, but we can do a wonderful job of needlessly worrying about ridiculous things, even to the point of making ourselves really sick.

Sometimes we blame our illnesses on things like the weather, germs, contagion, allergens, and even plants like poison ivy. If your attitudes are positive enough, nothing can invade your body. Every illness is nothing more than a negative feeling or belief manifesting. If you fail to make the Self-correction you need to make and go on with your negative beliefs, your health problems and energy imbalances will continue. You have to learn to say "NO!" to your negative thoughts.

I had an interesting experience with poison oak while I was taking training as an energy healer with The Four Winds Society. We were meeting daily at El Capitan Campground, about a fifteen minutes' drive north of Santa Barbara, California, along the coast. Each evening I would drive home about 10 o'clock, rather than stay at the campground, because I lived in Santa Barbara. At this particular time I was taking two weeks of training in a row, and we had only the weekend between classes.

During that first week as an exercise in shifting energy, we were required to draw a sand painting on the ground at the campground. A sand painting is a way to influence Spirit Energy to change something in your life. First you draw a circle on the ground with a stick and then create a picture of your life using natural objects (sticks, stones, plants, flower petals, or whatever is available) to depict characters, events, or objects. When you first create the sand painting, the arrangement shows the way things are now in your life. Then you rearrange, remove, or add stones or other objects that represent things you want to change in your life to create a new scenario to impress Spirit Energy with this new visualization. The campground at El Capitan is beautiful, with dense natural growth everywhere, so I was able to gather many natural objects to depict characters and events for my sand painting.

After one week of class I was at home on the weekend doing my laundry from the past week and was getting ready to return the following week. As I was loading my washing machine, I realized that I had a rash on the back of my left hand that was beginning to itch like crazy. I didn't have to think twice about what it probably was–poison oak! Rather than scratching it, I spoke directly to it and said "NO WAY! NOT TODAY!" Those little red itchy spots felt like ants crawling on my skin, and it was clear to me that they were eager to race up my left arm and cover me with rash. I continued to speak directly to them, and I said, "NO! ABSOLUTELY NOT! THIS IS MY BODY, AND YOU ARE NOT WELCOME HERE!"

This intense itch persisted for about two days, but I always met it mentally with total resistance, and I won. It finally gave up and went away. I washed all my clothes, went back to my training the following week, and had no further problems with anything growing at the campground. Learn to say "NO!" when *anything* tries to invade your body. When I first saw those itchy red spots on the back of my hand, if I had said, "OH NO! I HAVE POISON OAK," what do you think would have happened? If you claim it, you've got it. Attitude is everything.

The same is true with contagion. If you stop believing that you can catch an illness from another person, it will stop happening to you. If fear enters the picture, and you allow it to take you down, then enjoy your illness! In epidemics, fear runs rampant, but as long as you keep your thoughts and feelings positive and have no fear, you will not contract the illness even if you live in the same house with a sick person.

Several years ago I had a neighbor who knew no boundaries. We lived on the back part of a cul-de-sac, and there was only a short open fence between our backyards. The neighbor would put cat food and water through the fence into my yard, because my yard had better access to the big field behind our homes. Her intention was to feed any stray animals that might be roaming in the field. As a result, every cat in the neighborhood and every stray animal in the field, including three very large wild raccoons, were coming into my yard to get her food. The raccoons really scared me, because they would stay right outside my back door at night.

Each morning about 9 A.M. I would go out on my deck to feed my two cats, Bodi and Muffin. Muffin had wandered into my yard shortly after I moved in there, and I had adopted him because he was so thin and obviously a stray. These two cats *were* my family, since my children were grown and, except for them, I lived alone. This worked very well until my neighbor started intentionally feeding my cats at her house about 6 A.M. because she said they were hungry. So when I went out at 9 A.M. to feed them, they were nowhere to be found! Some days I would hear her calling Muffin into her yard in the middle of the afternoon to feed him a special treat. It got to the point where Muffin was living in her yard more than in mine, and I was getting angry!

One day a black and white stray cat found the neighbor's food in my yard, moved onto my deck, and did not leave. I did not want another cat. By this time the three raccoons had become a dangerous threat to me, so I called a company that catches wild animals to come and remove them from my yard. That cost me $350. I called Animal Control about the black and white cat, but they would not take him until I got shots for him. That cost me $35. Then I wrote the neighbor an angry letter and put up a six-foot fence. That cost me about $1,000. Then my neighbor stood in the street and had a loud angry fit about my fence.

Shortly after that my tooth started to hurt deep in my gums. My dentist said an oral surgeon was the answer. I called the oral surgeon. He said he would charge me $1,200 for a root canal. At that point it was very clear to me what the neighbor had been doing, but what was I doing? I was *chewing her out*! Once I saw my own negative attitude, I knew why my tooth was hurting. So I stopped finding fault with her, put my house up for sale, and moved out. Several months later I sent her a beautiful floral centerpiece for her Thanksgiving table. I never went to the oral surgeon, because after I corrected my own negative attitude, the pain vanished. Releasing pain requires Self-correction. That's all! Where is your pain?

Illness happens only at lower levels of thinking. At higher levels of thinking, there is no illness, but only positive thinkers can reach higher levels. You can think your way right out of an illness by lifting and improving your thoughts consciously and by discarding the negative words you've been thinking. You can also lift your thoughts by thinking the word "LIFT" over and over. If you are struggling with an illness, you need to rise in conscious elevated thought. Your negative attitudes and feelings have to change and reverse before an illness can disappear, and you can achieve this.

Dr. Wayne Dyer said on Oregon Public Broadcasting that after he was diagnosed with leukemia his children started bringing him printed medical definitions of what happens to you as you progress in leukemia. Leukemia is a malignant disease and can be fatal. So he said to his children, "I wish you wouldn't do that!" Why would he not want his children to put medical information in front of him? He knew that what happened to him was up to him. He said to his Creative Energy, "I AM WELL." He knew that he had to think the outcome he wanted and not get swept away by the doctor's negative diagnosis. He had also gone through a painful divorce, but he knew that if he thought at a higher level his illness would disappear. Be aware of your feelings all the time. Are you moving your energy in a positive or a negative direction?

MIND GAMES

Playing Mind Games is a fun way to reprogram your mental patterns. In these games you work inside your mind on your mental screen with your eyes closed.

Word Destruction

In Word Destruction, you take negative words apart in your mind until the remaining letters either spell nothing at all or become a harmless positive word. With your eyes closed, imagine the alphabet strung out like a clothesline up high in your mind. Now visualize the word FEAR in the middle of your mental screen in capital letters. Then lift the letter F right out of the word and put it on top of the letter F that's in the alphabet above. Now what does the word spell? EAR. Is that a negative word? No, it isn't, so now the word is harmless and will not influence your Creative Energy. It does not matter which letter (or letters) you remove as long as you destroy the negative word. You can remove as many letters as you want.

This is a good game to play if you find yourself worrying about something that hasn't happened yet. FEAR is a powerful negative word, and destroying it in your mind can prevent something negative from happening. Practice destroying your own negative words.

Mental Trap Shoot

Imagine yourself standing in the middle of your mental screen, holding a shotgun. Instead of shooting at clay pigeons that fly up into the air as in a trap shoot, you will shoot at negative words to blow the letters apart. You can decide ahead of time which negative words you want to work on, maybe even write them down on a piece of paper in front of you, or else just imagine the words as you play. When you say "PULL," picture the negative word flying up suddenly on your mental screen as you fire your shotgun and blow it into tiny pieces. See the letters scattering in all directions so there is no longer a word that spells anything. Repeat with each word you want to destroy. More words to practice on are: INSECURE, MISERY, LONELY.

Negative Word Clearing

This is a way to test yourself to see whether a positive or a negative word is in control in your mind at the moment. By consciously *adding* powerful positive words to your mind daily, you can purify your blood chemistry and protect your health. You can refer to the chart called, "The Word Was God," to practice clearing negative words from your mind. First say a positive word out loud, like HARMONY, and visualize it on your mental screen. Then watch to see if the positive word holds on your screen or if the opposite negative word, DISHARMONY, rises up from your deep mind and appears on top of the positive word. If the positive word is in control in your mind 51 percent of the time, which is what you want, the negative word will not appear on your screen. If the negative word DISHARMONY rises up when you're thinking HARMONY, say "No more DISHARMONY. I FEEL HARMONY!" Likewise, if you visualize the word HAPPY and it stays on your screen, then that is the way you feel, but if the words SAD or GRIEF appear, then the negative word is in control, so you need to *add* and *hold* the word HAPPY in your mind to bring the positive word back into balance in your thinking. Reverse negative words instantly in your mind until the positive word holds on your screen. Notice the feelings in your body as we go through this clearing exercise.

Close your eyes. I will say a positive word. You repeat that word out loud, project it onto your screen, and watch to see if it holds there. If a negative word comes up, reinforce the positive word by saying it out loud several times. The first word is VICTORY. The next word is POWER. The next word is COURAGE. Go through the same process by thinking other positive words. We want only positive words in our mind for positive outcomes. You can open your eyes.

A-Z Alphabet Game

As an Energy Being, you are made of the finest substance in existence. Using each consecutive letter of the alphabet, use high-level positive *feeling words* to describe who and what you are as pure Spirit Energy. Let yourself go as high as possible with your defining words. For the letter X, you can use words that begin with "ex" like EXCELLENT. Begin by saying "I AM" followed by your high-level definition of your Self, always advancing through the alphabet. If you are in a group, you can take turns and go around the room. Examples: AMAZING, BLESSED, COURAGEOUS, DIVINE, ENERGIZED, FORGIVING, GREAT.

8 STEPS TO SPIRITUAL UNFOLDMENT

PERCEPTION – *"OBSERVATION WITHOUT BEING CONSCIOUS OF YOUR OWN EXISTENCE"*:

1. You are totally unaware of yourself. You just look out at other people.
2. You believe what you see and hear out in the world is real.
3. You do not love yourself because you don't know you have a Self.
4. You look at your bank account to see how much YOU are worth (and it's not much).
5. You believe you are human and subject to human beliefs (you're old after 50).
6. You blame other people for things that go wrong in your life.
7. You can easily see what others are doing wrong, and you try hard to get them to change, but you make little or no effort to correct yourself.
8. You allow other people to upset you. You seldom control your emotions, and you have many health issues.

APPREHENSION – *"LEARNING AND GRASPING WITH THE INTELLECT":*

1. You begin to notice your-Self as well as other people.
2. You become aware that you are creating your own experiences as the reflection of your own thinking.
3. You begin to consciously love other people, but loving your-Self is believed to be selfish and conceited, so you don't do that.
4. You find by raising your sense of your own Self-worth, your bank account reflects greater value in exact proportion.
5. You may still think you are human, but you realize you are free to think about your-Self any way you choose.
6. You begin to understand that Your Thinking Causes for you, so rather than blaming other people for things that go wrong, you make an effort to think in a more positive manner.
7. You begin to change and improve your own negative feelings to positive feelings consciously, especially your feelings about your-Self, in spite of what other people are doing.
8. If someone upsets you, you endeavor to correct your own attitudes by being more patient, more tolerant, and more loving to everyone, including your-Self.

COMPREHENSION – *"UNDERSTANDING OR BEING UNDERSTOOD FULLY WITH THE INTELLECT":*

1. You know your-Self as the thinker, and you know what you think now creates your future experiences.
2. You stand at a higher level and observe your-Self thinking and projecting everything in harmonious, perfect ideals in spite of what the world shows you.
3. You realize you attract people into your life who reflect your own sense of love or abuse of your-Self, so you begin to love your-Self a lot more.
4. You understand that the more you love and value your-Self as unique and special, the more money naturally flows into your life.
5. The word *human* means "higher than the animals but lower than God," according to Webster. You realize that word does a poor job of defining someone like you, who is able to cause with his thinking.
6. You endeavor to consciously improve and lift every thought you think because you begin to understand and experience that your own thinking moves the Energy of Creation.
7. You begin to take Self-correction very seriously, and you work diligently on improving your own attitudes and disposition.
8. You realize you are the person who needs to stop thinking that something is always wrong. If you think that, you create that. You find your health improves greatly as you concentrate on improving your own attitudes. You learn to live in peace with your-Self.

USE OR APPLICATION – *"To Diligently Put Into Action. To Practice with Devotion"*:

1. You think of your-Self as Creative Light Energy or Pure Spirit Energy.
2. You USE your energy and mental powers to create whatever you want by opening your mind to it consciously.
3. You wisely know if you intentionally think the words "Self-Love" often, you will brighten your own auric light, and will prevent your-Self from ever experiencing depression or suicide.
4. You praise your-Self often by saying, "Good for me!" and it reflects as great abundance and security in your life. Jesus made Himself equal with God, and He could work miracles and manifest instantly. You have to decide what you allow your-Self to be "equal to."
5. You know you are made of Light Energy and water in the form of a temporary body that is controlled by the positive and negative thoughts you think each moment. You know the words you think regulate the chemicals in your blood.
6. The Spirit Energy you are made of obeys you to the extent that you believe in your-Self as able to move it without doubting your ability.
7. You know from experience that you are the only person you can change and correct.
8. You know the Creative Light Energy that you are made of reads and responds to your feelings, so you monitor your feelings carefully, so you understand your-Self very well.

CHAPTER SEVEN

RELEASING YOUR PATTERNS OF PAIN – THE ENERGY TREATMENTS

Everything in existence is the result of a pattern, from the clothes you wear to the foods you eat. A pattern is an original or a model for creating more of the same thing, and it can only create the same experience or form over and over until the pattern is changed. We have all seen the beautiful patterns of a rainbow in the sky, and maybe even a double rainbow. They can be breathtakingly beautiful, with their vast array of colors blending into one another. When you're looking at a rainbow, you know you're not looking at a tornado, because that pattern is different. The rainbow instills awe, wonder, and a moment of repose for us, while the tornado may instill fear and a sense of danger if it's close enough for you to see it. The night sky is full of star clusters in many patterns with various names–Orion, Andromeda, Virgo, for example, each named after a mythological person, animal, or inanimate object. Some patterns that we can see represent things that evoke our emotions, such as the Nazi swastika, the Star of David, or a picture of a cancer cell.

In addition to patterns that we can see, there are also many patterns that are invisible, like patterns of thought. These can only be seen as we learn to monitor our thinking. If you repeatedly react to someone with anger or irritation, you program your energy to automatically react that way in the future. For instance, while I was married, my husband and I would sit down for breakfast on Saturday morning. I would say something to him, but there would be no response, because he was reading the newspaper and holding it high, and he was losing his hearing. Yelling was not an option for me, so I would feel like I was eating alone. This happened repeatedly, to the point where my pattern of anger would kick in automatically the moment I sat down for breakfast. I wanted some company, conversation, and attention, and I was not getting any. Finally I realized how I was reacting, so I said to myself,

I CANCEL THE NEED TO REACT WITH ANGER AND FRUSTRATION.

After saying this a few times to myself with the right intention in my heart, I was able to sit at the table in silence and eat my breakfast in peace. You cannot expect the other person to change to please you, because they probably won't or can't. You do have to be aware of your own negative attitudes and work on your own self-correction to control the patterns of behavior you are creating with your habitual negative thinking.

Dr. Alberto Villoldo, founder of The Four Winds Society, said that the fuel that energizes a pattern is held just inside the luminous skin of your aura. When you react emotionally to someone or something, your negative emotions trigger the energetic fuel to dump the related negative pattern into your chakra, and you mentally experience that feeling and event again. For example, if someone has done something to you in the past that frightened or upset you, from that moment on, every time you think of that person, you will feel that fear or upset, just as if it's happening all over again.

Trillions of different patterns are captured in seeds, and every kind of vegetable or fruit grows from a seed with a unique pattern. We know we cannot grow a carrot from a cabbage seed, and we cannot grow a head of lettuce on an apple tree, because the pattern is specific to the seed. We know that as long as a seed is in its package, it will not grow; however, when it is planted in a garden in dark moist soil and given water and sunlight, the seed is infused with life, and the pattern begins to unfold and grow.

In everything that grows, the seed is in itself, and that includes in people. According to George Lamsa, author of the book, *Idioms in the Bible Explained*, a *garden* metaphorically is "a wife, a family." At the moment of conception, the seed or pattern that creates a man or woman child is planted in a dark moist place (the womb) where it receives water and nourishment until it's ready to be born into our world. A man without offspring, according to the Bible, leaves no seed. So we create more of ourselves from a built-in system of patterns contained in seeds.

If you have a picture taken of your aura, you will see how you look as a Spirit Being currently living in your body temple. You, as Spirit Energy, are Conscious Living Light. Your thinking causes this Light Energy to mold itself into various patterns and imprints. As you learn to control your energy by reprogramming and releasing your negative thought patterns, you become a conscious creator of your own experiences, rather than a victim of your negative emotions and long-held habitual patterns that are not serving you well. The Living Spirit Energy that you are made of will conform exactly to the shape of the patterns you create with your thoughts, words, and intentions.

The Inca knew how to change the patterns and shape-shift their bodies into various animals, birds, or trees and back again into their original form. As John Perkins says in his book, *Shape-Shifting Techniques for Global and Personal Transformation*, "How do you think Mayan pyramids were built, and the Egyptian pyramids, the great Incan fortresses, Persian temples, Easter Island, the Nazca lines, and on and on?" He says it could have been accomplished very simply if the secrets of energy transfer, shape-shifting, were understood. He explains that shape-shifting is a matter of letting one's energy body slip into another, combining with it. As elements of sin, evil, and various religious teachings entered our ways of thinking, the secrets of energy transfer were lost and forgotten. We no longer had the faith in ourselves that is required. We lost our courage and became afraid that we could not shift back into our own natural bodies. We have to recognize the difference between the SELF and the many golden idols that have stolen our power away.

Perkins says that those who shape-shift understand that all of life is energy, and that by focusing your intent you can change energetic patterns, rendering a new form. Shape-shifting can occur on three levels: cellular, transforming from human to plant or animal; personal, becoming a new self or leaving an addiction behind; and institutional, creating a new business or cultural identity. He says it's a matter of intent, faith, observation, and letting go of fear.

He also says that you have to know the difference between a dream and a fantasy. You want your dreams to come true, but if you give more energy to the fantasy, you may create what you don't want. You can empower a fantasy by fighting with it. It may not be possible to manifest your dream in the circumstances in which you are living. You may have to change your entire lifestyle abruptly to disempower the fantasy in its tracks.

Years ago a psychic told me that the themes of my life are death, money, and power. The death part of this lifetime has included losing my mother, my father, my sister, my husband, my two oldest sons, and the estrangement of my daughter, leaving me with only my youngest son, Douglas. The circumstances surrounding all their deaths and the estrangement of my daughter have resulted from Alzheimer's, alcohol and drug addiction, depression, suicide, and betrayal. When you find that everyone you have loved has died, including your children, it is so devastating that it disturbs your own life balance. As a result, I have dealt with grief, tears, anger, fear, despair, loneliness, and depression. If I had not had training in and access to the shamanic energy treatments that release these overpowering negative emotions, I would not have survived. These treatments give you a cleansing and a release from negative emotions that nothing else can even touch.

In The Four Winds training with Dr. Alberto Villoldo, each class is about five days long, from 8:30 a.m. until 10 p.m. daily with about an hour and a half for lunch, so it is very intensive training. As their student, you really feel like you're living in a different world where you can easily connect with Spirit, totally unlike our own world. I remember in Santa Barbara after I had taken two continuous weeks of their training in a row, I went to the beach by the Pacific Ocean and stood in the wind with my arms outstretched, trying to come back into this world, because their training is so different from the way we live.

The Four Winds teaches four modalities for healing. First, we learned the **Illumination**, which clears patterns or imprints from your luminous energy field. Second, we learned to **track and remove intrusive entities and energies** from the client's body, using crystals. Third, we learned the **Soul Retrieval**, where we journeyed into the past to discover an original wound, and the **Destiny Retrieval**, where we journeyed into the future to gain access to a possible healed state, as for a cancer patient, rather than a probable state. Fourth, we learned **Spirit Flight**, or the **Great Death Rites**. We learned to travel to the *hanaq pacha*, the *kay pacha*, and the *ukhu pacha*. Hanaq pacha refers to the upper world comprised solely of *sami* (the most refined energy). Kay pacha, the middle or physical world (Earth, Gaia), is the sphere of consciousness, ego, and identity (spirit made manifest), comprised of both sami and hucha (light and heavy energies). The lower world, *ukha pacha*, is composed solely of *hucha*. Hucha is heavy, disharmonious, and incompatible energy. It is not negative, bad, or dark energy, but is devoid of *ayni* (energetic cooperation).

CHAKRAS AND THE ENDOCRINE SYSTEM

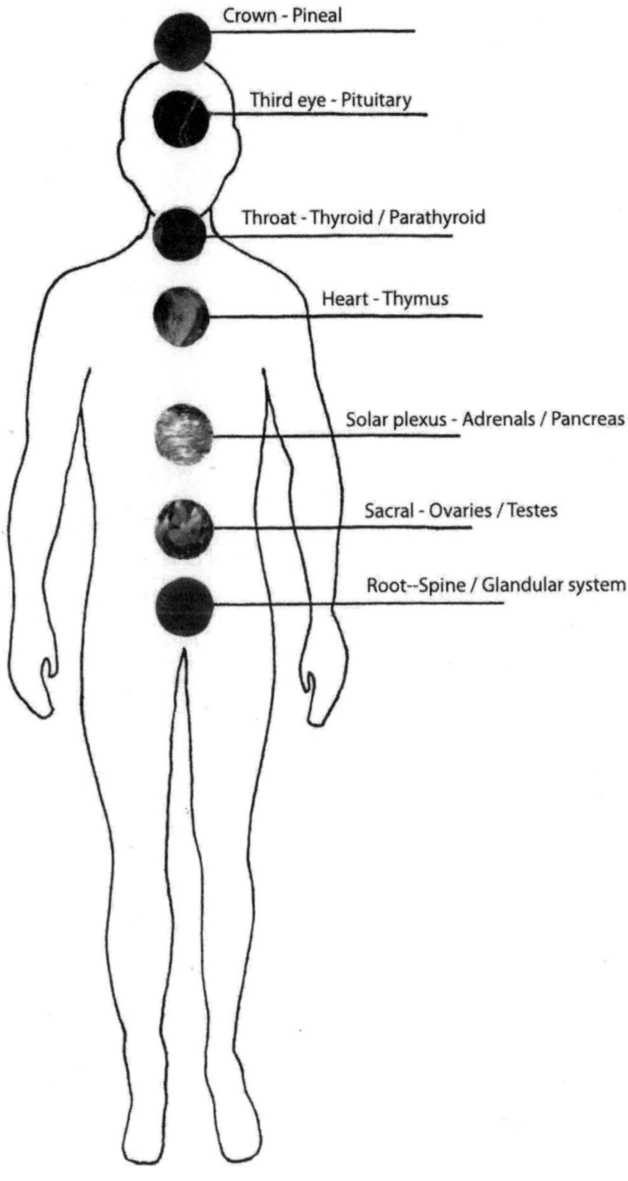

Dr. Villoldo teaches that there are four ways we process information through our chakras. The Medicine Wheel is represented by a Southern Cross (with equidistant beams). The names of the archetypes–Serpent, Jaguar, Hummingbird, and Eagle/Condor–refer to your chakras, starting with your root chakra.

THE MEDICINE WHEEL

ARCHETYPE	DIRECTION	ELEMENT	PROPERTIES
SERPENT	SOUTH	WATER	STONES, PHYSICAL, BODY
JAGUAR	WEST	EARTH	ANIMALS, MENTAL, EMOTIONAL, SYMBOLIC, WORDS
HUMMINGBIRD	NORTH	AIR	HUMANS, SOUL, MYTHIC, VISIONS, DREAMS, INTENTIONS
EAGLE/CONDOR	EAST	FIRE	PLANTS, PURE ENERGY, ESSENTIAL SPIRIT

The medical doctor uses the visible Serpent or physical level. The psychologist uses the invisible Jaguar or mental-emotional-word level. The energy practitioner/shaman works at all levels by (1) using the archetypes to read through the chakras, (2) by listening to the Spirit Guides, and (3) by using the Five Clairs to see, hear, feel/sense, smell, and touch whatever is being investigated.

The Five Clairs

Clairvoyance: Eyes – See
Clairaudience: Ears – Hear
Clairsentience: Hands – Sense/Feel
Clairalliance: Nose – Smell
Clairaubience: Tongue – Taste

THE ENERGY TREATMENTS

Dr. Villoldo says, "Every trauma that you have ever endured in any lifetime is etched into your aura like a blueprint. It holds the patterns for every disease you will experience, even years before it manifests in your body. It holds karma, ancient soul wounds, and pain. The fastest way to release negative energy and get your physical body to heal is to have an Illumination."

In the Illumination you enjoy a relaxing release of toxic energy from the *Luminous Energy Field* (your aura) that surrounds your physical body. It releases your negative patterns caused by trauma throughout time and space and frees you to handle your life minus the heavy emotions you've been dragging along through many lifetimes. Sludge is removed from the chakras using air, feathers, and hand motions. Rebalancing the chakras clears away the energy loops that make you susceptible to malignant physical and emotional conditions, erases imprints of disease before they manifest, and brings about healing at the blueprint level of your being. Crystals are used to extract invading energies or entities. Rips or tears in the luminous energy field are detected and repaired. Your aura needs cleaning monthly to keep it in prime operating condition. This treatment can be done in person, or at any distance by telephone.

1. **ILLUMINATION** – *clears imprints from the luminous energy field.*

When an Illumination is scheduled, I ask the client to fill out an Intake Form that gives me basic information about any chronic illnesses, injuries, pain, or special problems, and what he would like to release during the treatment. I ask him to wear comfortable clothes with no metals. If the treatment is done over the telephone long-distance, I ask him to be lying down and covered up to stay warm.

To prepare for the treatment, I open sacred space in my healing room to connect to the ecosphere. When the client calls me at the appointed time, I call in his energy with my intention, and it comes onto my healing table. Then I open the *noesphere* and place the *widacocha* over my client's energy and myself for protection in sacred space. I test his chakras for blockages, place a *kuya* (medicine stone) over the lowest blocked chakra, and alternately hold the deepening points and release points in the back of the client's head. Then I get out of the way, and the spirits come in and do the work. During the treatment I do a spiritual reading using the archetypes in my chakras. When the treatment is over and the client's chakras are clean and clear, I send the energy back to him, wherever he may be. This treatment takes about an hour and a half. Having an Illumination is like polishing yourself from the inside out so you feel a lot better, and your Auric Light shines much brighter. If you continue to have the treatments monthly, it purifies your energy at deeper and deeper levels.

2. **SEVEN CHAKRA ILLUMINATION** – *backwashes and removes intrusive entities and harmful energies from each chakra.*

This kind of reading is a mythological unfolding of your Soul's Journey through many lifetimes. I might find your Uncle John attached to your body, or I might find witches and demons in your chakras. This is not uncommon at all. One of my current clients is an American Indian from the Lakota tribe. When I performed a Seven Chakra Illumination on her, I saw her as an eleven-year-old Caucasian boy traveling west in a wagon train that was attacked by Indians. Everyone was killed, so in this lifetime she has come back as an Indian.

One story that has come up for me in two different readings is the tale of when I was a thirteen-year-old girl who lived in a medieval village, possibly in Germany, on the edge of a dense forest. The year was probably around 1200 or 1300. I was kind of a tomboy, and I usually hung out with boys around my same age. We all knew that the forest was a dangerous place, because there were lots of wild animals, but one day the boys were teasing me, and they challenged me to go into the forest because they knew it was forbidden. I took the challenge and went into the woods where I was devoured by wolves. I feel that all of that story has not yet been cleaned out of me, so it could come up again in a future reading.

In 1985, just five years after my son Michael's death, I was diagnosed with a tumor in my right ovary that the doctor said could be malignant. A tumor is caused from your feelings of guilt or remorse. I was still punishing myself over his death. I believed that good mothers do not lose their children. The surgeon that I employed removed a large benign tumor from my right ovary, but he left the red-hot energy that created the tumor in my body, because surgeons cannot see the invisible energy that causes the problem.

Twenty-two years later, another Four Wind's student and I exchanged Seven Chakra Illuminations just to practice. Two days later I had just returned home from the training in Park City, Utah, when the red-hot energy that caused my tumor in 1985 suddenly shot out of the right side of my abdomen like a rifle bullet, burning my organs as it came out. It took about three months for that burn to heal. I asked myself later whether, if I had known that the Seven Chakra Illumination would release red-hot energy that would burn me as it shot out of my body, would I have chosen to have that treatment anyway? Yes, I would. I am thankful to have that negative energy out of my body where it can never hurt me again.

How valuable is a treatment that can remove the pattern that causes cancer? No matter what your problem is, if you go to an Energy Practitioner first, you may find that your problem will disappear, and you can avoid surgery altogether. If you have surgery to remove cancer from your body, but later the cancer returns, that is because the surgeon could not see or remove the invisible pattern that caused the cancer. A shamanic Illumination can remove the pattern, but you have to be willing to go through the healing process that it requires.

Medical practitioners use their eyes to look outward at things that are visible: CAT scans, x-rays, blood samples and skin tissue; an Energy Practitioner/shaman uses her chakras to look inward at things that are invisible: visions, patterns, intentions, archetypes, and mythological symbols. A medical practitioner tries to cure the effects of negative energy gone wrong in the body; an Energy Practitioner cleans out the negative energy so nothing can go wrong.

A few years ago I had a female client in her fifties who

told me that when she was a little girl, probably about nine years old, her father gave her to his poker buddies as the prize for the winner. One of these poker buddies had died, and rather than ascending, he had attached to her body. In the middle of her Seven Chakra Illumination, I was commanding him to come out of her body when this entity said out loud through her mouth, "I'm not coming out." She heard him talking through her mouth and yelled back at the entity, "You ARE coming out!" But he continued to refuse saying he had won her in a poker game and she belonged to him. So I challenged this sick entity to a game of poker, and he accepted. After a moment I told him I had four aces. I said, "She's mine! Get out!" With that, his luminous body came out of her physical body into a crystal, and I escorted him to the Upper World. This kind of attachment is common. Many people we meet have entities or relatives attached to them without their knowledge.

Once I get the entity or relative into the crystal, an angel usually appears to help me take the etheric body of the relative to the Upper World. Working in dark mental space, if I hook my arm through the relative's arm the angel will often hook through his/her other arm so that the relative is in the middle as we fly through dark mental space to the Upper World.

Dr. Villoldo says that sometimes psychic objects that get into your auric field harden like petrified wood and become embedded in your physical body. They can take the shape of daggers, arrows, spears, knives, darts, wood, metal, or even glass, and may cause a lot of pain in your body. These psychic objects may have been thrown at you by someone who was angry at you, or you may have been angry at yourself and turned your anger inward. This kind of object requires a Crystallized Extraction because the pain stays in one place.

One day a beautiful blond lady came to see me for a treatment. She was experiencing atrial fibrillation and pain in her upper spine. I gave her an Illumination and discovered a psychic dagger with a black and silver handle in her heart chakra. The dagger looked Arabian, with a blade that curved up between her shoulder blades to the exact point where her pain was hurting. I extracted the psychic dagger and her pain was relieved. She was married to an Armenian man, and they were having marital problems.

If you feel a pain moving around in your body, this kind of negative energy requires a Fluid Extraction. A few years ago a man came to see me who had undergone surgery for an aneurysm in his brain. It was obvious that he could not function in a normal manner. Using my psychic vision during his Illumination, I observed a thick black substance extending from his heart up into his head. I opened his crown chakra and this substance began gushing out from the top of his head like a long flowing rope.

3. **SOUL RETRIEVAL** – *journey to the lower world (ukhu pacha) to discover an original soul wound.*

In a Soul Retrieval, I journey to the Lower World on your behalf to ask Archangel Huascar, Guardian of your Soul, to show me what will make my client whole, or to give me information about a particular problem. I usually take my spirit animals, Jaguar, Black Panther, Winged Lion, and the Angel, along to assist me. Within each one of your four soul chambers, I can see, hear, smell, touch, and sometimes taste whatever is there, and I listen to my spirit guides. In every chamber I look for healed soul parts to bring back to you, parts that have splintered off during traumatic events in your soul's journey through many lifetimes.

Chamber of Wounds – I may see an event where someone has harmed you, so I clean it out of your heart chakra with my crystal. If you are in depression, I may encounter demons that will attack me if they see my light, so I wear black to cover my light. My crystal is my flaming sword that captures them and protects me, so I carry it in my right hand.

Chamber of Promises / Soul Contract – If you have made a contract with Spirit in a past life, it may be hurting you in this life. It can be changed or torn up. An example that Dr. Villoldo gives involves a woman with twin babies living in a war zone. They are in a bombed-out building in freezing weather. She knows they will all be dead by morning. She says to Spirit, "Please let my babies die before I do." She wants to take care of them as long as possible. In her current life, her daughter was dying of cancer. By having a Soul Retrieval and removing this old Soul Contract, her daughter recovered.

Chamber of Passion / Grace – This is your purpose in life; it's what you're here to teach. There may be a Treasure Chest in this chamber. What appears in the chest reflects your own value of your-Self. The chest could hold rocks, marbles, hairpins, gold coins, diamonds, rubies, trash – or, nothing at all.

Chamber of Treasures / Gifts – I might see almost anything in this chamber. It could be a recap of things that were in the other chambers with deeper insight, or it could be new information. Spirit may give you a gift to help you in life.

Power Animal – Offers wisdom and assistance for you. When I come back from the Lower World to the Middle World (Ki Pacha) where we are, I bring back your healed soul parts and any gifts you have been given and blow them into your heart chakra. After the Soul Retrieval is complete, you go through a Sacred Drama where you ask the characters that appeared in your soul chambers why they were there and what they have to tell you, in order to get deeper understanding and clarification. You may hear answers that are deeply buried within your mind. Some people can hear these deep answers in their mind, while other people are not in touch with their inner voice at all.

Years ago I received a beautiful thank-you letter from a lady named Margaret. She wrote to thank me for helping her nineteen-year-old daughter. Margaret told me that Susie had been raped when she was twelve by an older teenage boy. Since that time she had been uncontrollable, belligerent, and difficult for her parents to live with. Margaret had taken Susie to many counselors over the years but had found no relief for her problems. Susie was talking about moving to Hawaii with her boyfriend and was not at peace with herself at all. In the Sacred Drama, Susie closed her eyes and asked one of the characters that appeared in her Soul Retrieval why she had been raped. After a moment of silence and inner listening she said out loud, "Punishment." Then she became quiet and thoughtful. She had done something at age twelve or younger for which she believed she deserved punishment, so she attracted to herself the abuser who fulfilled her belief. At the end of her Soul Retrieval, a white dove had appeared as her Power Animal, bringing back her purity and innocence. When I told her that Spirit gave her back her purity, it turned her life around, and Margaret wrote me that thank-you letter. For children who have been raped, their innocence and purity have been stolen from them, so the Soul Retrieval can restore what was lost.

While I lived in Santa Barbara, I had a dear friend named Marilyn. At that time we were both single, so we would go out to dinner, or see a movie or just have fun together. Earlier she had been in a difficult marriage. She was afraid of her husband, so in order to leave him she packed her car while he was not at home and drove away. I met her in a class we were taking, and we just hit it off. She was a very capable business woman who made a good living as a hair dresser. She also made and sold jewelry.

I had moved from Eugene, Oregon, to Santa Barbara, to be near my mother, who was dying from Alzheimer's when we met. As time went on, Marilyn became very active at Unity Church, and met a man who played guitar there with other musicians on occasion. She really liked this man, but he just wasn't interested in her romantically. Marilyn was a little heavy-set, so she started swimming every day in an effort to lose weight. She was a fabulous cook, and loved to have parties now and then in her apartment. But as time went on, she really wanted this man to love her, and he just wasn't cooperating.

I knew that my mother, at age 97, had reached the point where she couldn't visit with me at all, and it was just a matter of time until she passed away. I had done all I could do for her, so I made the decision to move back to Eugene, Oregon. Several months went by and I called Marilyn to see how she was doing. She said she had a lump under her arm and she didn't know what it was, but that she was feeling okay. I told her I was coming to Santa Barbara to visit my mother, and asked her if I could stay with her over the weekend. She said yes.

While I was there I asked her if I could give her a Soul Retrieval to see what was going on with the lump under her arm. She had told me she was going to see the doctor on Monday, the day after I was leaving. In the reading I did for her, I saw an angry dragon shooting fire and a little yellow canary teetering on a branch, trying to hold on. It seemed to be saying how fragile life can be. I left early Monday morning to catch a plane, and spoke to Marilyn later that week. She said the doctor told her she had cancer. Eight weeks later Marilyn passed away.

Since that time I have done a Soul Retrieval for a young woman in Eugene who had a tattooed dragon across most of her body, not visible when she was clothed. As I was doing her reading out loud, the spirit guide said to her, "If you bring the dragon to life, do not expect to live." At that point, the young woman lifted her blouse and showed me the large dragon tattooed across her body. She was being hateful to herself because she felt somehow responsible for her younger brother's death. He had been born with a physical impediment. I told her about Marilyn, and how I had seen the dragon before in a reading and how my dear friend had died. I told her that if she wanted to live, she had to stop being a beast to herself in her Self-talk. You cannot hate yourself and be well. It is required that you speak and act lovingly to yourself all the time to stay well, because your Self-talk is programming your Creative Energy to create the experiences in your coming moments. You cannot be a beast to yourself and survive. As far as I know, this young woman is still alive and, I hope she took seriously what I told her.

You have to treat yourself in a sweet, kind, and loving manner every moment of the day and night. You have to treat yourself with mercy and loving kindness. You have to remember that every moment you are alive is a privilege, a blessing, whether or not your life is going the way you want it to go. You have to learn to be content and to live in peace with yourself. You cannot be impatient or resentful, or try to run the world yourself, and still get along well. You can always improve your own thinking. You can be grateful for what is good in your life, and always hope that difficult things will improve, and THEY WILL as you improve your concept of SELF. The words you're thinking and the feelings you're feeling are creating your life every moment.

OTHER ENERGY TREATMENTS

4. SPIRIT FLIGHT / GREAT DEATH RITES

The Great Death Rites are performed on a person who has just died to free his or her spirit from the physical body. For a person who has not died, your luminous body is separated for a few minutes from your physical body, and you experience out-of-body spirit flight at the speed of light, because you are made of Light Energy. It helps you overcome your fear of death. Some people don't want to come back into their physical bodies because it is so freeing, but the magnetic pull is tremendous as long as the silver cord remains connected at your navel.

5. LEVELS OF ASCENSION

Another special treatment is the **Upper World Reading** (*hanaq pacha*). You have the opportunity to communicate with a departed loved one or friend whose energy is brought into the body of a surrogate.

One evening three ladies came over to have an Upper World Reading. Two of them were sisters, and their brother had been murdered several years earlier. They wanted to ask him, who killed him and discover any other information about his death. The third lady who came had agreed to be the surrogate to receive his energy. I told the sisters before they came to write out a list of questions they wanted to ask, because their brother's energy could stay here for only a few minutes. During the reading they asked him many things about his death, and he answered through the surrogate. By the time the sisters left they felt they had gained valuable information to go forward with an investigation.

When I bring anyone down into a surrogate, I take him back to a higher level than where I found him, if possible, although if he is still working through his issues, he may not be able to stay at the higher level.

Once you start having energy treatments, it's important to keep having them, because we go deeper into your negative energy with each cleaning. If you are going through an emotional time in your life or feel like you're coming down with something, that's a great time to have an energy treatment. Often these treatments will give you more relief than anything else you could do.

CHAPTER EIGHT

ILLUMINATION VS. INVASION

LET YOUR LIGHT SO SHINE

Climbing up, reach for the sky
Higher than high, see – I can fly
You say you can't! Did you ever try?

~Nancy Lynne Harris

Alcoholism, drug addiction, depression, and Alzheimer's are all caused from the same thing–the individual's unintentional neglect and ignorance of the Spirit nature of the Self. We live in a spiritual universe that we do not recognize as such, even though we are in the midst of a fierce spiritual battle that has been going on for centuries. Every time another person commits suicide or otherwise dies from dysfunction, the enemy has scored another victory. We, in our ignorance, just go on in the same old way, allowing this to happen over and over again. Winning spiritual battles requires conscious Self-awareness and willingness to change the failing status quo.

Complete healing from dysfunction is accomplished

only when the individual is willing to change from within and work on improving his Love/Hate relationship with the Self. We all know that dysfunctional illness cannot be healed with medicine. We must consciously recognize our responsibility for the CORRECT USE, rather than misuse, of the Light Energy we are each made of as Spirit-beings.

One day I was having lunch with three ladies. The one sitting directly across from me said she worked in a mental institution as a psychiatrist. When someone mentioned to her that I am an energy healer, she said to me in a disparaging tone, "Oh, you do woo-woo!" I said "No!" I was surprised by her condescending attitude, and I wanted to say, "What I do works, and I do not incarcerate anyone," but I did not say anything else. If your mind is closed, you will not save people's lives no matter how many graduate degrees you have. Our mental health system is failing. Albert Einstein said, "The definition of insanity is doing something over and over in the same way and expecting different results."

According to current national statistics, more than 70 percent of American families are now considered dysfunctional, with substance abuse addictions involving alcohol, drugs, and untreated mental illness. More teens are killed by alcohol than by all illegal drugs combined. Millions of people who drink are mentally ill.

A few years ago I ordered a catalog from the United States Printing Office in Washington, D.C., listing all the psychiatric providers and mental institutions in the country. They sent me a catalog as large as a Manhattan telephone directory. Why are there still millions of people with addictions and thousands of suicides each year if all these qualified psychiatric professionals are providing their services? Obviously, something is wrong here. Based on their current level of understanding, medically trained professionals try to solve spiritual problems in physical ways that do not work.

In depression, the doctor may give you pills to help you cope or sleep, but there is no magic pill to heal dysfunction. Even if you enter a treatment facility where you come out clean and sober, the cause of your problem is still present in your mind. Some patients are confined to mental institutions where they are sedated daily with drugs, sometimes for many years, with little chance of recovery. Suffering patients may even agree to have electric shocks and other archaic mistreatments administered by well-meaning people who do not understand the invisible cause of dysfunction. When we find that medically-trained professionals have done all they can and we are still ill, it's no wonder that we look for other modalities of healing. With millions of suffering people, we find the diagnosis of "medically incurable" unacceptable.

My dad Jack was a gentle, kind man, a chronic alcoholic, and a member of Alcoholics Anonymous. During my childhood, I remember him lying in bed sick and the doctor coming to our home many times to give him barbiturates to calm his nerves and a shot to help him sleep. Dad was so tormented, after many years of trying to recover from alcoholism, that he took prescription barbiturates while he was drinking, and his fourth wife found him face down on the floor, dead at age fifty-two. There was no relief for this poor man in spite of his many attempts to find help.

When I was about eight years old, I saw Dad sitting on the side of his bed one day. He said, "Nancy, come over here and sit down beside me. I want to share something with you." He opened the bedside table drawer, took out a copy of the Serenity Prayer and began to read it out loud to me.

God grant me the serenity
to accept the things I cannot change,
the courage to change the things I can,
and the wisdom to know the difference.

I will always appreciate my dad's gift to me that day. I wish with all my heart that I could say to him now, "Dad, I know what's causing your problem. I can help you get well!" He would be so grateful.

For many years the belief has been that dysfunctional people are abnormal. This belief creates so much shame and embarrassment that many suffering people do not seek help at all. How can anyone say that we are abnormal when there are millions of dysfunctional people? We have become the normal. We are the victims who are caught up in the dark energy affecting this world. Now it is time for us to come into the Light where we can see what is really happening so we can all get well.

The alcoholics or addicts that you may know could be your son or daughter or your wife or yourself, and they desperately need help. My son Michael was killed in a car accident in 1980, a few days after his eighteenth birthday. My son Jeffrey hanged himself in a state of depression in 2007. He was forty-eight with a nice wife and two teen-aged daughters. My ex-husband Ray died in 2011. He was experiencing chemical blackouts from alcoholic poisoning and many other problems. I have lost my family, but I will do my best to help you save yours. I know now that the purpose of my life is to teach you what is really happening in dysfunction so you and your family can get well. You can overcome addictions and even depression if you understand what the unseen underlying problem is. I will tell you how to recover from alcoholism, drug addiction, and depression based on Jesus' teaching. I know from my own experience that His method of healing works perfectly.

The event that changed my life was Michael's death. He was driving home at 6 a.m. from a drug party on a curving river road when he crashed our truck into a power pole that broke in half, fell across the truck, and killed him.

As a responsible mother, I blamed myself for his death. I began to hate myself intensely. You just don't lose your children. Over the next eight years I experienced chronic depression. In depression you're dealing with constant mental torment. There is ***no*** peace in your mind. One of the counselors I saw sent me to a psychiatrist who prescribed various medications–Amitriptyline, Lithium, Mellaril and Xanax. The medicines caused so many side effects that I chose to stop taking them, except for Xanax. Port wine and Xanax were the ***only*** things that ever gave me any relief. After eight years of doctors, counseling, and medicines, my chronic depression had not improved at all, and my inner voice was encouraging me to commit suicide.

At that point I decided to do something I had never done before. I remember that I had painted my fingernails bright red that day to help me remember whose life I was trying to save. I could hardly concentrate on anything, because of the screaming voices in my mind. I sat down on my couch, covered my eyes with my hands, and intentionally looked inward for the first time in my life. I said, "What the hell is going on in here?"

I instantly saw five ghost-like creatures moving around in my mental space, seemingly right behind my eyeballs. They appeared to be planning their next treacherous maneuver to use on me. One of these creatures turned his head and looked straight at me. They knew I was looking at them, but I had taken them by surprise. Instantly they all hid in the dark edges of my mental space, and my mind went black. In a state of extreme mental turmoil, I reasoned that this must be what Jesus meant by evil spirits. From that moment on I knew that my mental space was being invaded.

Jesus encountered a wild man
who lived among the tombs.
Night and day he was crying,
and cutting himself with stones.
Jesus said, What is your name?
He answered, My name is Legion for we are many.

Mark 5:9

Webster defines the word *legion* as "an army of five-to-six-thousand foot soldiers."

Jesus commanded, Come out of the man!
The Legion of evil spirits pleaded with Jesus.
They begged Him to send them into the swine
that were grazing on a nearby hillside.
Jesus said, Come Out!
And the evil spirits entered into the herd of swine
that ran violently down a steep hill
into the sea and were drowned.
When the invaders were gone,
the wild man was in his right mind.

Luke 8:30

In this story Jesus tells us exactly how to heal dysfunction. **There never was anything wrong with this man's mind. His mental space had been invaded by evil spirits (demons), and his mind had been possessed.** (The word *possession* according to Webster means "to lose control of yourself.")

I decided to use Jesus' method of healing on myself, since nothing else was working. I reasoned that Jesus conversed with the intruders, and if I could hear them screaming at me, they could probably hear me screaming at them. I began yelling at them, "GET THE HELL OUT OF MY SPACE!" They were trying hard to get me to commit suicide, but I always chose not to take the action.

In addition to commanding them to get out, I began to say out loud, **"I BELIEVE IN MYSELF,"** and they began to object loudly. They wanted to keep me under their control, so I said to them,

I LOVE MYSELF TO THE DEPTH, BREADTH AND HEIGHT OF MY BEING.
I DISSOLVE THE NEED FOR THE NEGATIVE VOICE.

By saying this, I was beginning to reverse my **Self-hatred to Self-love**, and this began to make a BIG difference. In so doing, I went against what my dear well-meaning mother had taught me as a child. She taught me not to love myself, because she said it was conceited. In 2010, Mother died of Alzheimer's. In Alzheimer's your mind is completely captured by demons. They kill zillions of us that way every year.

When I told my counselor that I was yelling at those creatures in my mind and telling them to get out, the counselor said, "Don't do that! Don't do that!" I guess she thought I was just imagining the whole thing. By continuing to do it Jesus' way rather than the counselor's way, I got well. What I learned in those eight years of depression is that two psychiatrists and two counselors could not help me at all, even though one of the counselors told me that I had come to see her forty-nine times. If I had continued to do it the medical way, I would be dead. No one "out there" can heal you from depression. I began monitoring everything that was going on in my mind and consciously reversing my hateful thoughts about myself to loving thoughts. If you want to get well, you have to change the way you think about yourself from within.

**LOVE YOURSELF WITH ALL YOUR HEART,
SOUL, AND MIND.
IT IS THE ONLY WAY TO GET WELL.**

My hatred of myself over my son Michael's death had been so intense that the word *hate* seemed to regenerate itself in my mind automatically. I could not think of a word that began with "h" (like *hope*) because my mind would turn the word into the word *hate*. I finally spoke directly to the word *hate* and used sexually explicit words to dispel it from my mind so it could no longer use my Creative Light Energy to reproduce itself. I said:

**HATE IS GUTLESS, IMPOTENT, DISEMBOWELED
AND PERMANENTLY STERILE WITHIN ME.**

This worked perfectly to stop that word from regenerating itself in my mind. I began to consciously hold the word LOVE in my mind, which I had never done before. By thinking the word LOVE, I stopped the course of my depression, but by thinking SELF-LOVE, I reversed the flow of my Creative Energy, and I knew for certain that I was getting well. To heal any illness, you have to reverse your negative feelings.

As I continued to think I LOVE MYSELF, I was feeling better every day because I was thinking about myself in a new positive way. By thinking Self-Love, I was driving the invaders out of my mental space. As creatures of darkness, demons cannot live in an atmosphere of SELF-LOVE, because thinking the word LOVE brightens the auric light that surrounds your body. Your auric light, composed of beautiful rainbow colors, can clearly be seen if you are photographed with a Kirlian camera or special computer software. You can see the picture of my aura on the cover.

One night, lying in bed with my eyes closed, I observed a long procession of creatures dressed in black hooded cloaks carrying lighted candles, moving in single file going downward, leaving my mental space, as if they were attending a formal funeral procession. But I knew it wasn't *my* funeral, it was theirs. I had won. After they were gone, my mind became so quiet that I was experiencing complete mental peace. It took me eight months of persistent positive thinking to achieve my wellness from the day I first observed them. I was owning and protecting my mental spirit space for the first time in my life. I had proved that we, as Beings of Light, are more powerful than they are as creatures of darkness, and we can control them. They had to follow my command to get out of my space, and they could not stay in an atmosphere of Self-Love.

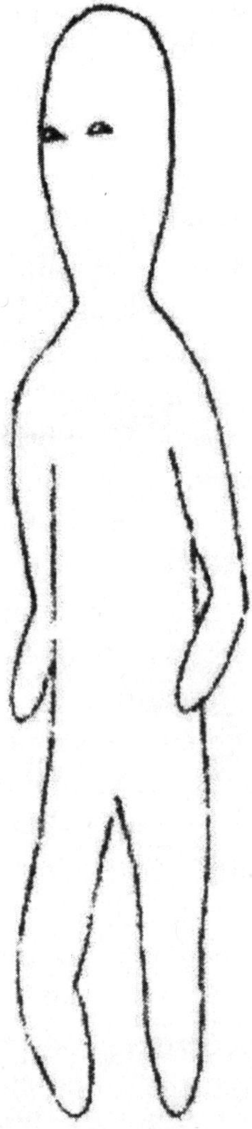

Evil Spirit – Demon – Fallen Angel
Sometimes they wear black cloaks.

James Van Praagh, the famous medium, says in his book *Ghosts Among Us*, "Individuals in an inebriated state are susceptible to ghostly attachment because alcohol depletes their protective auric field." He adds, "You would be shocked to know that many people who behave in horrific ways are being impressed or even possessed by dark and unevolved entities. They drain your energy and cause you to suffer accidents, injuries, and other misfortunes. Any form of chronic poor health can be a sign of ghostly attachment."

Drinking alcohol or using drugs creates portals (or what I call "space doors") in the luminous skin surrounding your auric field, enabling unevolved beings that live in dark immaterial spirit space to enter your individual auric field. These are dark entities that have lost the auric light THAT YOU ARE MADE OF, so they enter your mental space through these openings, or "space doors," that the alcohol and drugs create, and feed off your Light Energy. If you have an addiction, your mental spirit space has been invaded by these dark entities known as evil spirits or demons.

Actually, dysfunction is NOT an illness, and there is nothing wrong with your mind. This is why medicine fails to heal it. The mental space where your words form has been invaded and is under attack. In her book *Fallen Angels Among Us*," Elizabeth Claire Prophet calls these demons "extra evil." She says they are making a mockery of the paradise God created and intended for us here on Earth.

The ONLY thing that matters to you during a spiritual invasion is that you find relief from the intense mental torment they create. It doesn't matter how much you love your wife, your husband, or your children. All that matters to you is that you get relief. Usually alcohol or hard drugs are the only substances that numb you enough to provide any alleviation from the extreme mental torment you are enduring. A drug, whether prescription or recreational, is still a drug, and it helps to keep the portals open in the auric skin that surrounds your luminous energy field, so using drugs of any kind could prolong your addiction or depression.

The best ANY prescription drug can do is help you cope with the invasion that is in process in your mind, but medicine cannot touch or remove the invaders. Medicine goes into your body. The invaders are *not* in your body and *not* in your brain; they have invaded your mind. Your brain is an organ in your body. Your mind is *not* an organ in your body. It is where your thoughts form in spirit space. The mind is invisible unless you look inward. It is immense like the sky at night, and it would not fit into a brain.

DEMONS CAPTURE THE MENTAL SPIRIT SPACE WHERE YOUR WORDS FORM.

ONLY LOVING WORDS YOU THINK ABOUT YOURSELF CAN ENTER YOUR SPACE TO HEAL YOU.

THINKING "I LOVE MYSELF" IS THE BEST MEDICINE YOU WILL EVER TAKE.

Most of us are not taught as children that our mental attitudes, either positive or negative, reflect as our health, so when we are sick, we may feel that we are the victims of circumstances that we have no control over, but we are now looking at *our own negative attitudes as the cause of all illness with amazing results.* We know that negative attitudes are loaded with feelings, and your negative feelings can reflect on your body as illness.

To recover from alcoholism, drug addiction, or mental illness, you have to consciously choose to entertain the attitude of positive love and goodness toward yourself and others at all times in every thought you think and every action you take, and work diligently to achieve that goal. Most people believe they can think anything they want to think and it won't hurt them. That is a *grave* mistake. If you dwell mostly on negative thoughts, especially about yourself, you will create negative experiences for yourself, because YOUR THINKING CAUSES YOUR EXPERIENCE. If you drink, use drugs, and hate yourself, the demons will enter your auric field, take control of your thoughts and your life, and eventually encourage you to commit suicide. Many people die by their own hand every day. Once the demons invade your mental space, they *add* negative words to your thinking that you may not even notice at the time. Then you wonder why things are not going well in your life.

Demons possess our bodies to perform mass murders in "Batman" movies and in our public schools, such as Sandy Hook Elementary School in Newtown, Connecticut. Then we blame it on guns (something visible) and send hate toward the National Rifle Association because we are not suspecting an invisible enemy, and anything science cannot see is just a theory anyway. Of course, anyone suggesting that "demons did it" would be laughed at and called crazy by people with closed minds, so nothing meaningful is accomplished or changed, and the demons go right on killing us. Most "normal" people are really not paying attention to the problem anyway, in spite of millions of dysfunctional people among us, and most people in high places who could make a difference are not trained to read spiritual energy and don't understand it. Along with science, they think seeing is believing, but our invisible enemy can only be seen by looking inward, and science doesn't do that (that's woo-woo!), so no progress is being made at all toward ending the killings. This is the world we live in, and this scenario goes on and on around us all the time.

The Book of Enoch is an ancient scriptural work written before the third century B.C. that tracks antiquity back to the first hint of corruption upon a pristine Earth. This book was banned from the Old Testament and from the Hebrew Bible by the early church fathers, but it is part of the Dead Sea Scrolls discovered around 1945 in Qumran, which proves that the Book of Enoch was in existence before the time of Christ. It speaks from that obscure realm where history and mythology overlap.

The early church fathers agreed that the origin of evil was rooted in the angels who fell from heaven. The main subject of Enoch's prophecy relates to The Watchers, evil angels who were cast out of heaven and stripped of the Auric Light that identifies Spirit Beings as representatives of goodness, because of their lust for the women of Earth. The chief evil angel, Shemihaza, caused two hundred angels to bind themselves with a horrific curse, and with him they descended to Earth and mated with the daughters of men. Their progeny was a race of man-eating evil giants (who were destroyed by the Great Flood) and evil spirits. The fallen angels taught their women sorcery, incantations, and divination. They taught men every species of iniquity, including how to make swords, knives, shields, breastplates, and other instruments of war. Elizabeth Claire Prophet says that The Watchers, together with the progeny of the Nephilim–fallen angels who were cast out of heaven by Michael the Archangel–have continued to live on Earth without interruption for at least half a million years. Now the evil spirits invade our auric field whenever our portals are open to feed on our auric light like parasites and torment us until we commit suicide or die in some other tragic way, which millions of us have done.

How much longer will our scientists, our doctors, the people in power, and other enlightened intelligent people on Earth ignore what the evil spirits are doing to us? This is not a fairytale. We cannot go on living in ignorance any longer. As Like Attracts Like, so the level to which man has descended in consciousness is a magnet for any consciousness vibrating at the same low level.

Beholding your-Self and others in Love and Spiritual Perfection through Self-Awareness is the *only* way to elevate your consciousness to a higher level where evil spirits cannot enter your auric field with your death as their intent.

Whether or not you believe it, we are living in a Spirit World in a mythological story. We do not suspect our addictions or depression to be from a mental invasion caused by the negative way we think about ourselves or by our failure to recognize the Self as anything significant. S.E.L.F. is an acronym for *Scientifically Evolving Life Force.* Made of Spirit Energy, *we*, as GodSpirits, are the most magnificent beings in existence, and we treat ourselves so badly in our Self-talk that we create our own hell to live in. The Ancient Alien Society has a DVD for sale through the History Channel that deals with this topic, called *Ancient Aliens, Season Two, Angels and Aliens,* which I highly recommend.

Demons are translucent like clouds, even ghost-like in

appearance. They come in many shapes and forms just like we do. When they get into your mental space, they plan treacherous plots to terrorize and torment you relentlessly. They take control of your thinking, manipulate your inner visions, and raise the volume of your inner voice to loud, even blaring. They know what terrifies you because they can read your mind, so they play on it. They take control of your thoughts and use your body to perform heinous acts against other people, and use your mouth to speak hateful words to people who love you. They destroy your relationships. They invade the chambers of your soul. They hide in your blind spots (just like while driving), because they know you never look directly behind your eyeballs.

They use your children to do their killing in schools and homes. They have killed zillions of us over the centuries. They cause the wars where we kill one another and encourage us to kill ourselves. Trillions of us have committed suicide. The demons' goal is to capture and control enough mental territory so that evil will reign on Earth. Through recessions and years of war, they have been making headway, but there are thousands of us learning to brighten our auric lights by filling ourselves with Self-Love and Self-Praise, which is our best defense against their on-going invasion. The demons represent the direct opposite of what we are supposed to support–love and goodness in every thought we think about ourselves. Only the quality and quantity of your Love for Your-Self prevents these assassins from penetrating your energy field right now.

HATING YOURSELF CREATES MENTAL TORMENT.
LOVING YOURSELF CREATES MENTAL PEACE.

When we watch videos showing the universe, we can clearly see both light and dark energy in space. Each kind of energy has living beings that represent that energy. Each kind of being lives in the same universal mental space, some representing the light, some representing the dark. We, as Spirit-Beings, represent positive Light Energy, with our beautiful auric light shining from us. The evil spirits, who represent dark energy, know that we are the GodSpirits, otherwise they would not spend so much time and effort invading and killing us.

We don't know yet how this Battle of the Spirits will end, but you are playing your part in this conflict with every thought you think. If you swear at yourself and call yourself names, you are supporting the negative and keeping yourself open to invasion. If you choose to support positive love and goodness toward yourself and others across the board, then your urge to drink or use drugs will gradually disappear, you will get well, and you will help to heal this world. When 51 percent or more of the people on Earth collectively brighten their auric light by Loving the Self, the positive shift on Earth can happen. Until then, we will continue to experience a combination of some good and some evil. We have to choose to support love and goodness individually and collectively to enable Love and Peace on Earth to manifest.

I did not learn what I have shared with you here from reading a book or taking a class. I write from first-hand experience. After I saw the evil spirits in my mind by looking inward, it was just a matter of deductive reasoning to figure out how to get rid of them, and I succeeded completely. Now, as a Shaman and Spiritual Teacher, I extract demons from my clients with energy treatments, and I work to educate people as to the cause of dysfunction on Earth. We can turn this around, but not if we go on in the same old ways that are failing. You will help to save the lives of millions of tormented people on Earth who will otherwise die if you do your part to LOVE YOUR-SELF and SPREAD THE WORD.

HEALING MENTAL INVASION

1. PROTECT YOURSELF–USE YOUR EYES TO LOOK INWARD OFTEN.

If invaders have violated your space, you can see them if you look quickly. They are ethereal, transparent and cloud-like, and they do not want to be seen. They are completely evil and will torment you until you commit suicide. You can see their eyes looking back at you before they hide in the shadows.

2. LOVE YOUR ENEMIES.

Send love to the evil spirits in your mental space to drive them out. They cannot live in an atmosphere of love. I SEND LOVE TO THE EVIL SPIRITS IN MY MENTAL SPACE. GET OUT! THIS IS MY SPACE!

3. LOVE YOURSELF.

The amount of Love, or God-consciousness, you have for your Self determines whether or not evil spirits can enter your mental space. The word LOVE held in your mind will stop the course of mental invasion, but Self-Love will drive the invaders out of your mental space. Say, I LOVE YOU, (your name) often.

4. PRAISE YOURSELF.

Self-Praise is the greatest protection you can give yourself. Praise yourself for noticing every little thing that you can improve and think better. Say, “GOOD FOR ME,” often. The object is to get Self-Love and Self-Praise rolling in your deep mind when you are not thinking about them so they will always protect you. I PRAISE MYSELF. GOOD FOR ME.

5. RETRAIN YOUR NEGATIVE SELF-TALK.
Always monitor what you are thinking. Tell your negative inner voice that you do not answer to what it just called you. Then tell it what endearing name it may call you by. If the voice says anything objectionable to you, just add NO MORE to that thought, so you instantly reverse the negative thought to positive. Call yourself by an endearing name now.

6. BELIEVE IN YOURSELF AS BECOMING GREATER EVERY DAY.
Jesus made himself equal with God. He could manifest anything instantly by commanding energy perfectly. We can learn to do this, too. I BELIEVE IN MYSELF. I think only positive loving thoughts about myself.

7. GIVE YOURSELF PERMISSION TO CHANGE.
Healing requires self-correction. You have experienced what negative thinking has done for you. Reverse all your negative words to positives. I AM WILLING TO IMPROVE MYSELF. I CAN CHANGE.

8. FORGIVE EVERYONE. Do not harbor the negatives. Let it go. Move on.

9. LIVE IN PEACE WITH YOURSELF.
No fault-finding. Fault-finding reflects on your own body as faults. This means no swearing, no yelling, no kicking, hitting, ripping, stabbing or otherwise mentally abusing

yourself in your Self-talk. Peace and stillness is your mental goal. Self-persecution and Self-destruction must stop.

10. TEACH YOUR CHILDREN TO LOVE THEMSELVES.

It is never too late to tell your children to love themselves. You may prevent them from becoming dysfunctional, and you may save their life. Self-Love and Self-Praise are the greatest protectors of all.

11. SAVE A FRIEND. TELL HER (HIM) TO LOVE HERSELF.

12. REMEMBER THAT YOUR THINKING CAUSES.

Jesus said, "The Father and I are One." The Father IS the Creative Light Energy that you are made of. Use your energy wisely.

BALANCE OF ENERGY

Shadow/Negative	***Light/Positive***
Poverty	**Prosperity**
Invasion	**Protection**
Imbalance	**Balance**
Disease	**Health**
Mental Torment	**Mental Peace**
Self-Hate	**Self-Love**
Addictions	**No Addictions**
Nothing	**Magnificent**

100%

\+ *Indecision* - 50%

0%

Balance of Energy Chart

CHAPTER NINE

CASTING YOUR NET – WHAT ARE YOU WORTH?

Give a man a fish and you feed him for a day.
Teach a man to fish and you feed him for a lifetime.

A *miracle*, according to Webster, is "An extraordinary event manifesting the supernatural power of God fulfilling His purposes; an event or effect in the physical world deviating from the laws of nature; an accomplishment or occurrence so unusual as to seem beyond human capability or endeavor."

In the beginning, the miracles you work do not have to be instantaneous. When you have mastered the techniques, like Jesus, then you can work instant miracles. While you are learning to be a master, the object is to get the energy to change or reverse so that you manifest what you do want or something close to it. If you can believe in yourself enough to create the change you want even little by little, then you are at the kindergarten level of working miracles, and that is wonderful. So it will take some experience and practice on your part to become an instant miracle master, just like learning anything else worth learning.

To work a miracle, you must understand the exact negative-feeling word you need to change and then reprogram your energy by reversing that word in your mind to the exact opposite positive-feeling word. Remember, your success in working a miracle is proportional to your persistence in thinking the opposite positive-feeling word without faltering or giving up. If you stop short of your goal and decide it's not going to happen, then you have made a negative choice, and it stops the process. To work the miracle, you have to believe in yourself as able to do what you're trying to achieve. Your Self-confidence will grow as you begin to experience success in healing simply by changing your mind.

In spiritual terms, everything is in levels, from lower to higher. You are now living at the level of the words you have been using to describe yourself. As you consciously brighten your auric light through Self-love, you will naturally rise on the spiritual elevator, so eventually you may be able to help other people rise and get well by teaching them to love themselves.

Manifesting money is not about where you work or how you invest. There are many books written about both of those subjects. Your money is the reflection of your own sense of Self-value. It is relative to how you compare yourself to your concept of God or Spirit, whatever the highest concept of spiritual greatness is for you. Many people live their whole lives and never even know they have a Self, much less that it has to be valued to produce wealth for you.

In my work as an Energy Healer and Shaman, I often perform Soul Retrievals for my clients. One of the things I may see in the client's third soul chamber, the Chamber of Passion and Grace, is a Treasure Chest that looks similar to a pirate's chest. It's usually about eighteen inches long and twelve inches wide. The contents always tell me how this client values him or herself. Sometimes I see gold coins, emeralds, rubies, or diamonds in the chest, which indicate that this person has high Self-value. More frequently in the chest I see piled-up whiskey or wine bottles that are mostly empty with a few sticky drops left in the bottom. The corks are out, so liquor has spilled here and there in the mess inside the chest. In one reading I even saw hatpins and hairpins inside the chest, which indicated that this woman had no Self-value at all.

In a Soul Retrieval, I often find psychic manure (or dung) usually in a client's first soul chamber (the Chamber of Wounds), but if it also appears in the Treasure Chest or in other chambers, it means that this person spends serious time using profanity. Swearing at yourself or using God's name in vain creates psychic manure in your own soul chambers. You carry this psychic manure around with you on your soul's journey through many lifetimes until you have an energy treatment to clean it out, so it creates much impurity in your luminous energy field (your auric field). Keeping your energy clean and pure is one of your goals for success in healing. The words you think and speak create your life.

**SELF-LOVE CREATES YOUR HEALTH.
SELF-VALUE CREATES YOUR WEALTH.**

Your money reflects what you believe you deserve based on who you think you are and how you feel about yourself.

So by answering the following questions, you can evaluate your beliefs to increase the flow of money in your life.

1. **WHO ARE YOU? I AM…** (Make a list. Write it down.)

In "The Gospel of Thomas" from *The Gnostic Bible*, Jesus says:

Seek and do not stop seeking until you find.
When you find, you will be disturbed
Then you will marvel and rule over all.

In the third verse, He says:

The Kingdom is inside you and it is outside you.
When you know yourselves, then you will be known,
And you will understand that you are children of the living father.
But if you do not know yourselves,
Then you dwell in poverty and you are that poverty.

Notice here that Jesus says you have to know your-*Self* as who you really are, not as who you thought you were. You have to become aware of how you define *Self* now so you will be able to change that definition into a higher concept of who you really are. Before you can know yourself, you first have to recognize that you have a Self. Remember, the word SELF is an acronym that stands for:

SCIENTIFICALLY EVOLVING LIFE FORCE

(This definition was given to me by my
Spirit Guides many years ago.)

Jesus said, *My burden is Light*. You know that energy, as Light, produces reflections or shadows. You, as Children of Light, *are* the Light Energy reflecting your own mental conceptions and beliefs. Energy, as *sami* (golden light), is the most refined perfect prana, but as *hucha,* it is heavy or dense. Elevated righteous thinking is your goal to keep the *hucha* out of your body, bank account, and life.

Jesus understood that Living Light Energy, or Spirit, was the substance of His being. That's why He called it Father. Your Energy, your life-breath, is the Father, the substance of everything, awaiting your next proclamation. Your breath is Living Light or Spirit. When we speak lovingly and non-critically, we create more love. When we speak hatefully or angrily, we create more hate. We move the energy we are made of with our breath and our words, so we are moving the energy all the time.

Jesus said, *Cast your net on the right side.* The word *cast* as a verb means to "send forth by throwing," like throwing out a fishing line, but *cast* as a noun means "to give a particular shape by pouring liquid into a mold, or to yield or bring forth." A mental pattern, therefore, is like a cast that brings forth your net. The word *net,* of course, is a money word, which brings us to the next question.

2. **WHAT ARE YOU WORTH AT THIS POINT IN YOUR LIFE?** (Write it down.)

How did you determine your value? Did you consider the balance of your bank account to determine what you are worth? Do you value yourself in dollars and cents? Your bank account cannot reflect what you are worth. It only reflects a mistaken sense of your real value. Only you can evaluate your own Self-worth, and as you do, your bank account will perfectly reflect the level you choose. But if you look at your bank account to determine your Self-worth, you are starting wrong. **Never look into the material world to assess your value.**

Remember, you came from a God seed–a seed that grows Gods. How valuable is that? Re-evaluate yourself. Raise your conception of Self into the world of Spirit, which means you are Spirit Energy. There is nothing higher than what you are. You are it! Jesus made Himself equal with God. He and God were one. He knew He was made of what God is. He worked instant miracles. Learn the lesson. Go and do likewise.

Who is doing the thinking in your mind? Think as God would think. What you believe is what you get. If you're not getting what you want, lift your thought by lifting your concept of Self. Your sense of Self-worth programs the Creative Energy, or Spirit, to provide for you exactly what you feel you deserve, no more and no less. If you believe you are human, that is a certain level of Self-value. If you believe you are Creative Light Energy, or Spirit, you greatly elevate your sense of Self-worth. You can always change your beliefs and increase your wealth by raising your sense of who you are and what you're worth.

You communicate directly with Spirit Energy every time you think, because it is what you are. The Energy doesn't care which way you think, positive or negative. It will faithfully lift you high or knock you down based on the way you treat yourself in your Self-talk. Think about that next time you're down on yourself and turn your feelings around. Consciously lift yourself higher. Make careful choices in life so you can feel good about yourself, because you can really knock yourself out with your negative Self-talk. Always have goodwill toward Self and toward others. Be grateful for every good thing in your life. *Appreciation* is a money word that brings you more abundance just for thinking it.

The famous Chinese philosopher Lao Tsu said,

TO KNOW WHEN YOU HAVE ENOUGH IS TO BE RICH WITHOUT MEASURE.

He did not count his money to see how rich he was. Spirit Energy created unlimited wealth for him, because he knew that if he always said he had enough, he would always have enough. He did not put limits on his wealth. Do not allow yourself to think it or say it any other way, and do not doubt that the Creative Energy will produce for you, because it will always produce exactly as much as you believe it will. If you can understand that YOU are MADE OF pure Spirit Energy that is controlled by the words you think, then your bank account will always reflect an endless supply as you choose to think the value words that produce your money.

Do not limit where your money can come from as long as it's an honest source. Remember, making money is EASY. It's easy to move, easy to stand, easy to forgive, easy to get well, easy to make money, and very easy to love yourself. Think it right. Everything is easy. Money comes in easy. Money flows to you from everywhere all the time.

If you think of the word *prosperity*, *pro* means "to affirm, to favor, to support." *Esperit* was borrowed from Old French *espirit* (animating or vital principle, breath of life), and *spiritus* (soul, courage, vigor, breath) was borrowed into English directly from Latin. So *prosperity* means "for Spirit." If you are for Spirit, then you prosper because you are for your-Self!

We live in a spirit world where the Creative Energy reflects back to us whatever we think into it the most. You have to know where you're putting your mental energy, and pay attention to what you're thinking so you can Self-correct when necessary. Everything you need to produce money (or anything else) is built into your makeup as a natural part of you. You just need to learn how to use your spiritual equipment correctly.

In spiritual healing, we deal with our intentions and our imagination to visualize and dream our world into being. You have to think of yourself as pure Spirit Energy capable of anything, and let go of any negative ideas about your abilities. By believing in yourself as able and powerful, and by changing and improving words in your mind (in spite of appearances in the world), you re-program your energy to create a better outcome for you.

Your future moments will pay you dividends in exact proportion to the improvement in your thinking. What you think today becomes your experience tomorrow. The thought always precedes the event. You can always think something in a better, higher way. Think in perfect ideals to mold your Creative Energy into the most perfect outcomes possible. You can use your imagination to think as if you live in paradise, where you will have everything you need, because as the Creator, you will live wherever you think you deserve to live. Your thoughts enable you to create anything you can imagine. As long as you think something is wrong, something will always be wrong. There are no limits except those you impose on yourself.

Put off the former conversation,
the old man, which is corrupt...
and be renewed in the spirit of your mind...
put on the new man, which is created in righteousness.

Eph. 4:22-24

If you wanted to have your house appraised, you would contact a professional appraiser. He would look around and put a value on your home based on the location, size, amenities, and the market. To determine your own value, you are the appraiser. Your Self-worth has to be relative to something you're familiar with, so with each of the following objects, look into your mind and sense how you value yourself in comparison. Are you worth more than the item listed, or is the item worth more than you are?

1. a $50,000 bill
2. a diamond necklace
3. a new black Maserati
4. a champion race horse
5. a large cherry tree in bloom
6. an angel
7. the sun
8. water
9. your own child
10. your own reflection in the mirror

How does your value relate to these things? What are you worth?

YOUR MONEY AND YOUR BANK ACCOUNT REFLECT YOUR SENSE OF SELF-VALUE.

YOUR BODY AND YOUR HEALTH REFLECT YOUR SENSE OF SELF-LOVE AND MORALITY.

The third question is:

3. **"HOW DO YOU FEEL ABOUT YOURSELF?"** (Write it down.)

Dr. Alberto Villoldo says, "Self-awareness is essential if you're to serve in your role as Creator, because it means you're cognizant of your power to create as well as your power to destroy." He says, "Humility means being honest about what you are, so that you neither inflate nor underestimate your value. You recognize your intrinsic beauty and Self-worth and are comfortable with your gifts. Emptying the mind is the ultimate act of humility, because then you can be free even from your own preconceptions."

Your negative feelings about yourself have created the blockages, illnesses, and lack in your life that you are now experiencing. Maintaining perfection requires *moderation* in all things to keep your energetic balance positive–not too much, not too little–so think carefully about what you need to change for improvement.

To be born into the world of the Spirit, you have to become aware of yourself as a Spirit. The word *Spirit* according to Webster means "a special attitude or frame of mind." You have to monitor and control your attitudes, because your attitudes move your Spirit Energy. You will find yourself moving into greener pastures as you raise your sense of who and what you are. Remember, you are not what you appear to be. You are Light Energy (Living Spirit) camouflaged in a temporary body, as a picture of your aura will easily reveal.

There are three steps in the creative process. In religion it's called the Holy Trinity, but in reality it's not something to worship. It is the instruction manual for how to operate your-Self to create what you want.

YOUR SUBSTANCE	YOUR CHOICE OF WORDS	YOUR RESULT
LIGHT ENERGY	FEELING	FORM
BREATH	SELF-TALK	MANIFESTATION
POWER	ATTITUDES	REFLECTION

To consciously shift energy, you have to reprogram your Self-talk. This is the still small voice that goes on constantly in your mind. By persistently thinking and saying carefully chosen positive words, you can reverse a negative mental program created by your habitual negative attitudes in past moments to reverse an illness or a sick bank account. The words you choose must be the exact opposite positive *feeling* words from your former negative attitude about it. To reverse the energy, analyze your negative feelings and *add* the opposite positive words to your thinking. Repeat these words over in your mind many times a day to re-program your Self-talk in a new way of thinking that you are consciously choosing. When your thinking-balance of positive-to-negative words reaches 51 percent positive, the energy will shift and the manifestation will change–your bank account will increase automatically and/or your illness will vanish. Your health, wealth, and life will change exactly as much as you succeed in changing your Self-talk to positive across the board.

To reprogram, you have to watch yourself think. Look for the highest and best words to think about everything, and *add* them to your mind daily. Begin to use money words to inform your ever-present Creative Energy what you think you are worth. The Spirit Energy you are made of *is* the most precious substance in existence, so as you re-evaluate yourself, you are not lying to yourself. You are just getting to know yourself a lot better. Spirit Energy can create anything you want. You just have to open your mind to it.

I have found the phrase "no more" to be very effective in reprogramming old negative patterns. When you first notice yourself reacting in a negative emotional way, say out loud to yourself,

NO MORE FAULT-FINDING! NO MORE DISCONTENT! NO MORE IMPATIENCE!

Then *add* the exact opposite positive words to your thinking by repeating them out loud, even if it's not the way you *feel* at the moment to calm yourself down and avoid creating a new negative pattern. Your goal is to maintain your inner peace so you do not project negative energy inward. Tell yourself:

NOTHING IS WRONG. ALL IS WELL.

If you feel that something is wrong, your energy will continue to create something wrong, because that is what you are programming in. When you get upset, you are messing with the God/Spirit Energy because your energy *is* essential Spirit.

Faultfinding is one of the worst things you can do because it creates faults in your own body. Realize that your negative attitudes, patterns, and beliefs are causing your pain and illness. Negative energy in your body has substance, and pushes hard against your organs, trying to find a place to lodge. If you pray for healing, but make no effort to correct your negative attitudes or beliefs, your pain will continue no matter how many prayers you say. You control the energy that creates your pain. Self-correction is always necessary for healing.

Avoid using words that start with the letters "dis," like disharmony or distorted, because they will all be negative words. The exception is the word *dispel* meaning "to scatter or break up," which you can use to remove negative feelings when you are reprogramming your mental patterns.

NO MORE ANGER!
I DISPEL MY PATTERNS OF ANXIETY AND SELF-HATRED.
I LIVE IN PEACE WITH MYSELF.

Look for the good in everything and voice only that. Your goal is to keep your emotional state on the positive side no matter what is going on. When you consciously reverse your negative attitudes to positive attitudes, you can achieve your healing and overcome pain in your body. Conscious reversal of negative words in your mind moves the Creative Energy to heal your body.

You have to STOP judging (coming to negative conclusions) by the way the problem appears in the material world. You create the change you want by thinking and seeing everything as perfect (including yourself). You are not pretending when you think that way; you are reprogramming toward perfection. If you persist, you will achieve your goal.

Don Miguel Ruiz says in his book *The Voice of Knowledge*, "You are heaven's child." Stop thinking of yourself as "human" because that word is demeaning. Think of yourself as made of the animating principle of life. You have to stop misjudging yourself as the lowest of the low and claim your birthright as Creation's Master. There is nothing finer in existence than what you are, because you're made of Spiritual Light.

You have to learn to divide the chaff from the wheat, including religious beliefs from the truth of your being. God does exist, not as a deity to be worshipped, but as an entity to be understood. Our beloved idols die hard, but when you are born into a truer concept of SELF by rising above beliefs from the past, you will find that all you have to do to work a miracle is to change your mind. It requires no pills or prescriptions, and there's no expense–just intentional thinking at higher levels in spite of the way it seems to be by observation. When you become a positive thinker, healing becomes a do-it-yourself job. If people understood this, hundreds of millions of people would stop ingesting drugs of any kind, legal or illegal, that kill them. What a miracle that would be!

Close your eyes for a moment and ask yourself this question:

How does it *feel* to have complete control over the words you choose to think and the attitudes you choose to entertain? After you have pondered that feeling deeply, open your eyes and answer question four.

4. **WHAT IS YOUR VALUE NOW?** (Write it down.)

We all know that the universe is a complex subject. Even our most brilliant scientists can ponder unanswered questions for years before they arrived at a possible hypothesis. We know that the sun is the source of our light, and we take it for granted that it will still be shining there tomorrow. Without the warmth and power of the sun to grow our food and keep us warm, we could not exist. Our sun radiates with the same Light Energy that burns within each one of us as Beings of Light. We have to keep our own sense of love, purity, morality, and goodness burning within ourselves so the Light from the sun will keep shining on us and not grow dark from our Self-neglect.

Richard Panek, author of *The Four Percent Universe: Dark Matter, Dark Energy, and the Race to Discover the Rest of Reality,* which won the American Institute of Physics communication award in 2012, says, "Astronomers have compiled evidence that what we've always thought of as the actual universe–me, you, this book, planets, stars, galaxies, all the matter in space–represents a mere 4 percent of what's actually out there." He says that 23 percent of the rest of the universe the astronomers call "dark matter" and 73 percent they call "dark energy."

According to an article in *Smithsonian Magazine* from April 2010, "Scientists have hardly a clue about dark energy." Michael S. Turner, a University of Chicago cosmologist, has ranked dark energy as "the most profound mystery in all of science." While Light Energy is the warmest and most life-giving energy in existence, dark energy is the coldest of all substances, minus 100 degrees Fahrenheit, where life as we know it could not exist.

According to an article on Hubblesite.org, the fate of the universe is one of the many questions that astronomers ponder. When they realized that the universe is expanding at an accelerating rate, they also realized that it requires significant changes in our understanding of the way the universe works.

Whatever we see reflecting *out there* in the universe began as a thought *in here*, within the collective attitudes of mankind. By recognizing yourself as a privileged Being of Light choosing to support only the good and by perfecting your positive attitudes consciously each day, you will find that the energy in the universe will improve exponentially.

We are not born dysfunctional on this Earth, yet millions of people become dysfunctional while living here. Our over-crowded mental institutions and prisons attest to this. Dark energy actively wars against Light Energy in our daily lives even though we may not recognize this fact. We tend to blame dysfunction on the individual rather than on the true cause. We, as Light Carriers, have the power to turn the nightmare of dysfunction around, because the words we think individually control our lives, while our collective thinking controls the energy in the universe.

We know that we live in duality on this earth. The Light Energy and dark energy in the universe are reflecting our positive loving feelings and attitudes, as well as our negative hateful feelings and attitudes on a moment-by-moment basis. The dark energy in the universe is currently reflecting a much larger percentage of our negative thinking *(hucha)*, rather than our positive thinking *(sami)*.

The Bible says THE WORD IS GOD. The words that we think are controlling the universe. We have not taken ourselves seriously as Creators, but we need to wake up. Not only does our thinking create light or dark energy in the universe, the more we hate ourselves, the darker our individual auric light will become, which enables fallen angels (demons) to enter our individual auric field.

I, as a shaman, can see, hear, and extract these creatures by looking inward and by performing Soul Retrievals on my clients. I am not, by a long shot, the only person who is able to see the fallen angels. They can be seen by anyone who is able to look inward, and they are attacking us here on Earth big time every day. This has been going on for centuries because we are unaware and we are allowing it. Taking a pill to get rid of them is a joke.

There are millions of people who are alcoholics, mentally ill, depressed, drug addicts, or suffer from Alzheimer's. These people have indulged in negative thinking about the Self to the point where they have been invaded by fallen angels whose goal is their death. To overcome this problem, we need to monitor our attitudes moment by moment, thought by thought, or we will be in for a *grave* awakening as we approach 100 percent dark energy in the universe, which is the direction we are currently heading.

If dysfunctional people were taught to reprogram their energy by thinking *Self-Love* constantly throughout each day, they would begin to brighten their auric light and to get well. The invading demons would be forced to leave their auric field, because they cannot live in an atmosphere of light (thinking Self-Love creates Light). We have to learn this lesson to keep our children and ourselves healthy and alive and to begin to make some progress in solving this terrible invasion that is going on every moment we fall into negative thinking in this world.

The more we love ourselves, the brighter our individual auric light becomes, disabling fallen angels from entering our individual auric fields. Keep your Inner Light burning brightly by choosing to Love Yourself and to support the good in every possible way in your attitudes.

LOVE YOURSELF TO
BRIGHTEN YOUR AURIC LIGHT

I recently watched an awards show on television where celebrities in the audience were sitting there in their finery wearing horns attached to the top of their heads. As I observed that, I thought, what am I seeing here? Do these people even realize what they are choosing to support? The fallen angels are out for your blood and your God energy, because they lost their God light (unlike us) when they were cast out of heaven in antiquity (according to the Book of Enoch).

If you choose not to love yourself consciously, or leave it all to chance, you may open yourself to invasion by fallen angels who will create great dysfunction for you without your ever knowing why you can't stop drinking, using, or taking drugs.

When Jesus healed people, He *sent* His word to reverse the negative energy. To increase the Light Energy and decrease the dark energy in the universe, we must collectively and individually work to *send* positive vibrations of energy into the universe by staying positive in our daily thinking at all times and by understanding what we are supporting.

By collectively loving ourselves and keeping our attitudes positive across the board:

(1) Light Energy will gradually increase in volume at the individual and universal levels as a reflection;
(2) The expansion of the universe will begin to slow down rather than continuing to speed up until it explodes as is now thought to be a possibility;
(3) The new Light Energy we collectively create will expand throughout the universe and overcome the

dark energy as we use our abilities to love ourselves more as powerful Beings of Light;

(4) Collectively, we as God-Beings, are much more powerful than the evil spirits. We just have misunderstood who and what we are.

This is not something we can put off till tomorrow. Love your-Self today, tomorrow, and forever to help turn the world around now. Your ONLY opponent is your own negative voice. If our "failed mental health system" (as it has been called numerous times since the murders at Sandy Hook Elementary School and many other places) will not look at the invisible realities that exist and continue to blame dysfunction on our brain, lack of serotonin, and the NRA, then we will continue to die at increasing rates. THIS IS NOT ACCEPTABLE!

The cause of our problem is *spiritual neglect of the Self.* Everything in this world is "of Spirit," and reflects as either Light Energy or dark energy. There are no other choices. We have to choose which attitude we serve thought by thought, moment by moment, and start protecting ourselves consciously. You have to know what you are choosing to serve, support, and *invest in*. Every thought matters! You may just need to tweak your attitude a little to achieve the success you want and deserve to work your personal miracle. Remember, if you're not getting the miracle you want, you have not reversed your attitudes.

ATTITUDE IS EVERYTHING.

Be conscious of your thoughts as fresh unused Spirit Energy unfolding your feelings and thoughts exactly as you are choosing to think it.

Hunger and thirst after righteousness (right-mindedness).
Matt. 5:6

Joseph Campbell said, "Healing is what happens when we step beyond suffering into myth." We are living in a mythologically unfolding universe that we do not recognize as such.

Can we choose to support the goodness that we were born into in spite of the deceptions we are taught in this world? Can we come to understand the SELF in time to save our world from the direction it is now heading? Overcoming the fallen angels would be the miracle of the century, and we, as GodSpirits United, can achieve this.

Teach your children and everyone else to love themselves with all their heart and soul. The more you love yourself, the more you rise in spiritual elevation, and your own Self-Love will gradually open your inner door to the voices of your spirit guides who will answer your questions and guide you through life.

Seek and ye shall find.

Luke 11:9

Knock and the door shall be opened.

Matt. 7:7

From now on, practice thinking from the top down rather than from the bottom up. You ARE a Powerful Creator no matter who you think you are. Loving and praising yourself brightens your auric light and shuts the invaders out of your luminous energy field (your aura) forever. There is no other way to protect yourself in this world from the invisible forces and dark energy around us. If you want to keep the darkness out of your own auric field, you have to keep your Light turned on at all times.

LOVE YOURSELF WITH ALL YOUR HEART, SOUL, AND MIND.

So the last question is:

5. **WHO ARE YOU? WHAT ARE YOU WORTH?** (Write down your answers on the following worksheet.)

MANIFESTING MONEY WORKSHEET

1. WHO ARE YOU? I AM ____________________________

____

____

____

____

____

2. WHAT ARE YOU WORTH? ______________________

____

____

____

____

____

3. HOW DO YOU ASSESS YOUR VALUE? __________

____

____

____

____

____

4. HOW DO YOU FEEL ABOUT YOURSELF? ________

____

____

____

____

____

To manifest change:

1. *Empty Out*

   I AM CHANGING.

   I RELEASE ALL NEGATIVE ENERGY FROM MY MIND AND BODY.

   I RELEASE EXCESSIVE CLUTTER FROM MY HOME NOW.

2. *Fill*

   I FILL MY ENTIRE BEING WITH NEW, FRESH, PERFECT, LOVING, HEALING SPIRIT ENERGY.

3. *Reflect*

   MY BODY, MIND, AND LIFE AUTOMATICALLY REFLECT MY NEW PROGRAM WHEN I REACH AT LEAST 51 PERCENT POSITIVE THINKING.

Affirm moment-by-moment:

1. I LOVE MYSELF WITH ALL MY HEART, SOUL, AND MIND.
2. I HOLD TO THE PERFECTION OF MY BODY ALWAYS.
3. I AM PERFECT, WELL, STRONG, AND HAPPY IN BODY, MIND, SPIRIT, AND SOUL AT EVERY AGE.
4. EVERY DAY IN EVERY WAY MY LIFE GETS BETTER.
5. MY BODY AUTOMATICALLY REFLECTS WHAT I THINK MOST.
6. I AM SINGLE-MINDED ON THE GOOD BY CHOICE.
7. I MEDITATE DAILY, CONCENTRATING ONLY ON MY BREATH.

8. I CLEAN UP MY MOUTH AND NEVER SWEAR AT MYSELF.
9. I AM NATURALLY THE BEST OF THE BEST WITHOUT TATTOOS OR PURPLE HAIR.

Write the following words on all of the mirrors in your home so they reflect back to you:

SELF-LOVE, I LOVE MYSELF

Ye are the Light of the world.
Let your Light so shine…

Matt. 5:14-16

ABOUT THE AUTHOR

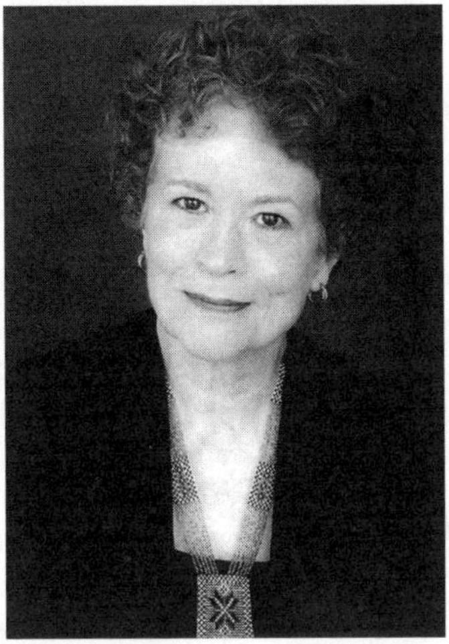

NANCY LYNNE HARRIS, M.A., is a graduate of The Four Winds Society, the world's most extensive professional training in energy healing and shamanism, founded by Dr. Alberto Villoldo. She was trained as a Spiritual Teacher by the Eschatology Foundation in Los Angeles. She completed advanced training in Theta Healing and was recognized by Worldwide Who's Who for excellence in energy medicine.

Nancy is the founder of GodSpirits United, LLC, a company formed to help people recover from medically incurable illnesses. She teaches that at the essential level we are each made of Light Energy. Through workshops, books, and CDs, she teaches you how to shift your energy to make positive changes in your health. Nancy specializes in helping people recover from alcoholism, depression and glaucoma.

To order other works by Nancy Harris:
www.GodSpiritsUnited.com or www.Amazon.com

Healing Alcoholism Invasion Revealed (tradepaper)

Heal Yourself of Anything Example Glaucoma (tradepaper or CD)

Consciously Overcome Mental Illness (spiral bound or 2 CD set)

How to Heal Your Hang-Ups – depression, alcohol, drug addiction (CD)